You don't have to be bored when you diet!

USE THE FINGERTIP
LOW CALORIE GUIDE

CHAPTER 15

to find out which foods are
200-350 calories
100-200 calories
50-100 calories
20-50 calories
20 calories or less

You'll find delicious surprises like these...

Under 20 calories:
1 dill pickle
1 cup spinach

Under 50 calories:
1 egg roll
1 cup popcorn

Under 100 calories:
1 extra light beer
4 ounces gefilte fish

Under 200 calories:
7 ounces beef stew with biscuits
7½ ounces macaroni and cheese

Under 350 calories:
13 ounces eggplant parmigiana
8 ounces oysters

Le Gette's *Calorie* ENCYCLOPEDIA

Bernard Le Gette

WARNER BOOKS

A Warner Communications Company

WARNER BOOKS EDITION

Copyright © 1983 by Bernard Le Gette
All rights reserved.

Cover photo by Frank Marchesano

Warner Books, Inc.
666 Fifth Avenue
New York, N.Y. 10103

 A Warner Communications Company

Printed in the United States of America

First Printing: January, 1983

10 9 8 7 6 5 4

Contents

Contents

Introduction

Losing weight is simple. It's not easy—but it's simple. You cut the intake of your calories, and then you lose weight. Everything else you've ever heard is icing on the cake you can't eat. Carbohydrates, cholesterol, volume, protein, metabolism, exercise, are all very interesting, and confusing, to think about, though none of these things plays a big role in how much you weigh or how little you can weigh.

But even when people cut calories they usually don't do a very good job of it. You have probably gone on diets, wondered why they didn't work and wandered off them again, or maybe they did work, but your will power collapsed—

the constant pressure of not eating so many delicious foods caved you right in.

There are two reasons why most people fail. The first is that they don't really know how many calories they're consuming. They estimate how many calories are in each food, estimate how much of each food they ate, and constantly say things like, "That was only a little snack—two or three crackers." Sound familiar? And of course they're always rejecting potatoes.

Well I'll tell you right now, there is no way you can estimate. You can't estimate the size, you can't estimate the number of calories and you can't estimate the number of times you snacked. You can't estimate a thing. You aren't that smart. Nobody is.

You have to count the pieces, weigh them, and check every time how many calories you just ate. And then you have to write it down. Every calorie. Every day.

Now I know this is more inconvenient than being fat, and hating yourself every day, and being tired, and having heart attacks. But that's the way it is. It does have the advantage of being one inconvenience instead of many, and it is also only one simple way to lose weight—instead of many complicated ways not to—which brings us to the second reason most people fail.

It's because losing weight tends to get very vague in people's minds. It's a hidden enemy that has to be strained against every day. And that's very disheartening—which means it won't work. Any constant general restriction on your life, that has no definite limits and no clear procedure, is just not going to work. That's why specific diets are so successful in the short term—they remove the vagueness, the guesswork, the doubt. But we aren't talking about the short term. We're talking about weighing whatever you like for the rest of your life.

Fortunately, you don't have to fight hidden enemies. You don't even have to use much will power. You only have to know how to count—calories.

The purpose of this book and the years of research that went into it is to give you—in one place—the calories of all the foods you might ever eat. Whether it's fresh, or a commercially packaged brand, or a meal you ate in a restaurant or prepared at home, or a snack you ate at a drive-in—it's here. The portions listed are as standardized as is practical, so you don't have to bring your calculator. There are no extra columns of things that won't help you lose weight, and there is as little repetition as possible. You won't find listings of Thingamajigs—25 calories; Thingamajigs on a stick—25 calories; Thingamajigs sliced—25 calories, and so on. If thingamajigs are 25 calories, that's all you need to read—very simple.

The chapters are in a logical order chosen to

help you remember where things are listed. If everything were listed alphabetically you wouldn't know if some fish would be found under fillet, or haddock, or Mrs. Paul's, and even when you found it you couldn't compare it to others of its kind. So everything is in these fourteen basic groupings.

And the fifteenth chapter is the Fingertip Low Calorie Guide. This is an innovation which I hope will enable you to find a variety of low calorie foods at a glance. They are listed in calorie groups so you can plan your shopping, your meals, even your snacks with a specific number of calories in mind. It is also a pretty thorough list of the low calorie foods available. As you'll see in the rest of the book, being called *low calorie* or *dietetic* is no guarantee that a food is low in calories.

Everything is listed for normal usage. That is, if a food is made from a mix, say, the quantity and the calories listed are for the food after it's been prepared according to the package instructions. Likewise, it is of no use to know how many calories are in a pound of spinach while it is still frozen, so that is not listed. Now some things are listed as containing 0 calories for one tsp, and that is accurate; it is also reasonably accurate for one tbs. I can't guarantee, however, that there are no calories in three lbs. of sweetener. There just might be a few.

So how do you lose weight? Eat *what* you want, though of course a balanced diet is always best. It's not what, but *how many* that counts. Remember, virtually all foods have calories. The question is, how much satisfaction and/or nutrition are you getting from a particular food? For the calories in it, a plain potato contains a phenomenal variety of nutrients— you can probably live longer on potatoes than on any other single food—and that would suit some people fine. Others, however, would like to go quickly on apples, which contain neither calories nor nutrients in any marked degree.

But however you do it—eat fewer calories. Measure every portion. It's quite easy. Just put your chicken, or your potato, on a scale, see what the scale says, and compare that to the portion listed in this book. Write down the number of calories for each meal. Add them up at the end of the day, and in the morning write down how much you weigh next to yesterday's calorie total.

But you have to do it every time. It won't do you any good sometimes. And if after awhile you think you can remember most foods' calories, you're wrong. You have to measure. You have to count. The reason you're fat (which is why you bought this book) is you don't know how to play it by eye. You were brought up to eat too much, your aggression makes you hungry, your metabolism is rotten, whatever. It doesn't matter. You want to be thin. I just told you how. If you really *want*

to be thin, that's what you'll do. Otherwise
you'll continue to play at it and make excuses.

Now if you want to look good and be
completely healthy *in addition* to being thin, you'll
also exercise, though the exercise won't do either
of those things for you if you're overweight. And it
won't help you to lose much weight either. The relation
between calories and exercise is straightforward.
The harder it is, the more calories you burn.
There are 3,600 calories in 1 pound of fat. Roughly,
you'll burn 100 calories by:

skating (either kind)	45	minutes
skiing (either kind)	35	"
football	30	"
handball	22	"
walking	19	"
rowing	18	"
bicycling	15	"
chopping wood	13	"
swimming	12	"
jumping rope	11	"
jogging	10	"
running	6	"

or (even more roughly) 18 holes of golf (on foot) or
two sets of tennis.

So if you want to lose that pound of fat, it's
easier not to eat the 3,600 calories than to jump

rope for 7 hours. What will help the most is a regular, steady approach to food and calories. This book can be your guide to help you look and feel the person you really want to be.

1 quart	= 4 cups
1 cup	= 8 fluid ounces (oz)
1 cup	= ½ pint
1 cup	= 16 tablespoons
1 ounce	= 2 tablespoons
1 tablespoon (tbs.)	= 3 teaspoons
1 jigger, or shot	= 1½ ounces
1 pound (lb.)	= 16 ounces

Remember, a fluid ounce is a measure of volume, not weight.

ALL listings are for food *as prepared* for normal usage. That means that after it's been prepared with all the normal ingredients, and it's ready to eat—that's what the calories are for.

CHAPTER 1

Beverages

SPIRITS, WINES, LIQUEURS, COCKTAILS, BRANDIES, AND COCKTAIL MIXES

Note: The number of calories in distilled spirits depends entirely on the alcoholic content—the higher the proof, the higher the calories. This is true for bourbon, gin, rum, Scotch, tequila, vodka, and almost anything called whiskey.

Distilled Spirits, 1 oz

80 proof	65
90 proof	75
100 proof	85
150 proof	125

Cocktails, canned or bottled, alcoholic, 1 oz

Amaretto Sour
Mr. Boston   40
Apricot Sour
Party Tyme   33
Banana Daiquiri
Party Tyme   33
Daiquiri
Hiram Walker   59
Mr. Boston   33
Party Tyme   33
Calvert   63
Gimlet
Party Tyme   40
Gin & Tonic
Party Tyme   28
Mai Tai
Lemon Hart   60
Mr. Boston   36
Party Tyme   33

Manhattan
  Calvert   54
  Mr. Boston   40
  Party Tyme   37

Margarita
  Calvert   59
  Mr. Boston   35
  Mr. Boston strawberry   45
  Party Tyme   33

Martini, Gin
  Calvert   63
  Hiram Walker   55
  Mr. Boston   33
  Party Tyme   41

Martini, Vodka
  Calvert   63
  Hiram Walker   49
  Mr. Boston   34
  Party Tyme   36

Old Fashioned
  Hiram Walker   55

Piña Colada
  Mr. Boston   60
  Party Tyme   32

Rum & Cola
  Party Tyme   28

Screwdriver
  Mr. Boston   39
  Party Tyme   35

1

Sour, Gin
Calvert   65
Sour, Scotch
Party Tyme   33
Sour, Tequila
Calvert   65
Sour, Whiskey
Calvert   60
Hiram Walker   60
Mr. Boston   40
Tequila Sunrise
Mr. Boston   40
Tom Collins
Calvert   65
Party Tyme   29
Vodka Tonic
Party Tyme   27
Wallbanger
Mr. Boston   34

Cocktail Mixes, bottled and dry, nonalcoholic, 1 oz or 1 premeasured packet

Alexander
Holland House   69
Amaretto
Holland House   79
Banana Daiquiri
Holland House   66

Mint Julep
Holland House 67
Old Fashioned
Holland House 9
Party Tyme 28
Piña Colada
Holland House 60
Party Tyme 50
Pink Squirrel
Holland House 69
Planter's Punch
Party Tyme 37
Screwdriver
Holland House 69
Party Tyme 21
Sidecar
Holland House 17
Sour, Blackberry
Holland House 50
Sour, Virgin
Party Tyme 50
Sour, Whiskey
Canada Dry 11
Holland House 53
Holland House low calorie 9
Party Tyme 29
Party Tyme instant 53
Sip 'n Slim
Holland House 10

1

Strawberry Sting
  Holland House   35
Tom Collins
  Holland House   58
  Party Tyme   44
  Party Tyme instant   58

Cocktails, standard recipe, alcoholic, 1 oz alcohol, unless noted

Bacardi	155
Bloody Mary	140
Brandy Alexander	225
Bourbon Highball (1½ oz bourbon)	
with soda	125
with ginger ale	180
Cuba Libre	224
Daiquiri	135
Gimlet	136
Gin Fizz	172
Grasshopper	235
Irish Coffee	214
Manhattan	177
Martini, Gin or Vodka	115
Mint Julep	209
Old Fashioned	144
Orange Blossom	153
Pink Lady	190
Rob Roy	199

1

Rum Cola (see Cuba Libre)	224
Screwdriver	168
Side Car	161
Sloe Gin Fizz	155
Stinger	149
Tom Collins	170
Whiskey Sour	142

Wines, 4 oz

Alsatian	
Wilm	88
Altar, red	
Gold Seal	132
Henri Marchant	132
Blackberry	
Manischewitz	180
Bordeaux	
red	
B&G Margaux	83
B&G Prince Noir	81
B&G Saint-Emilion	84
Chanson	108
Cruse	92
Cruse Saint-Emilion	92
Cruse Saint-Julien	92
Cruse Médoc	96
Cruse Château La Garde	108

1

 Chanson   108
 Gold Seal   85
 Henri Marchant   86
Cabernet Sauvignon
 Inglenook   77
 Martini   120
Capella
 Italian Swiss Colony   85
Catawba
 pink
  Gold Seal   132
  Great Western   148
  Henri Marchant   132
  Manischewitz   129
  Taylor   130
 red
  Gold Seal   128
  Henri Marchant   132
 white
  Gold Seal   132
  Henri Marchant   132
Chablis
 Gold Seal   88
 Great Western   92
 Henri Marchant   90
 Inglenook   76
 Italian Swiss Colony   89
 Taylor   98
Champagne
 Bollinger   114

1

Gold Seal blanc de blancs	98
brut	81
dry	91
Great Western brut	100
dry	104
pink	108
Henri Marchant blanc de blancs	88
brut	91
dry	98
Lejon	94
Korbel	104
Manischewitz	88
Mumm's brut	88
dry	111
Taylor brut	101
dry	104
pink	108
Veuve Clicquot	104

Chianti

Brolio	88
Gancia	88
Italian Swiss Colony	87

Claret

Gold Seal	109
Inglenook	80
Italian Swiss Colony	86
Louis Martini	126
Taylor	96

Cold Duck

Gold Seal	97

1

   Great Western   121
   Taylor   120
Concord
   Gold Seal   132
   Henri Marchant   132
   Manischewitz
      red   160
      white   130
      medium dry   120
      dry   85
   Mogen David   160
Kosher
   Manischewitz
      sweet   170
      medium   112
      dry   91
Labrusca
   Gold Seal   130
   Henri Marchant   132
Lake Country
   Taylor   106
Liebfraumilch
   Anheuser & Fehrs   80
   Dienhard   95
Malaga
   Manischewitz   180
Moselle
   Dienhard   95
   Julius Kayser   77

Great Western	96
Pinot Chardonnay	
Gold Seal	85
Henri Marchant	85
Louis Martini	120
Pinot Noir	
Inglenook	77
Louis Martini	120
Pouilly-Fumé	
B&G	80
Rhine	
Gold Seal	91
Dienhard	80
Gallo	67
Gallo Rhine Garten	78
Great Western	97
Henri Marchant	92
Julius Kayser	74
Inglenook	100
Italian Swiss Colony	86
Louis Martini	120
Taylor	92
Rhineskeller	
Italian Swiss Colony	88
Rice Wine	
Chinese	152
Japanese	286
Rhone	
Chanson	112

B&G 93

Riesling

Dienhard 96

Gold Seal 92

Henri Marchant 92

Inglenook 82

Louis Martini 120

Rosé

Cruse 96

Gold Seal 99

Henri Marchant 96

Italian Swiss Colony 86

Taylor 92

Sake 151

Sancerre

B&G 80

Sauterne

Gallo 67

Gallo Haut 83

Gold Seal 97

Gold Seal Haut 109

Great Western 105

Henri Marchant 109

Italian Swiss Colony 77

Louis Martini 120

Mogen David cream 59

Mogen David dry 39

Taylor 105

Soave

Antinori 110

Thunderbird
  Gallo   139
Valpolicella
  Antinori   109
Zinfandel
  Inglenook   76
  Italian Swiss Colony   80
  Louis Martini   120

Aperitif and Dessert Wines, 4 oz

Asti Spumante
  Gancia   168
Aquavit
  Leroux   300
Campari   66
  Dubonnet Blonde   151
  Dubonnet Red   190
Madeira
  Gold Seal   144
  Henri Marchant   144
  Leacock   160
  Sandeman   168
Muscatel
  Gallo   144
  Gold Seal   210
Pernod
  Julius Wyle   315

Port

Gallo	146
Gold Seal	185
Great Western	178
Italian Swiss Colony	170
Louis Martini	215
Robertson	180
Sandeman	184
Taylor	195

Sherry

Gallo	104
Gold Seal	185
Great Western	156
Taylor	200
Dry Sack	160

Sherry, cream

Gallo	150
Gold Seal	205
Great Western	180
Louis Martini	175
Taylor	178

Sherry, dry

Gallo	110
Gold Seal	162
Great Western	140
Italian Swiss Colony	132
Louis Martini	180
Sandeman	145
Taylor	152

Vermouth, dry
C&P	148
Gallo	100
Gancia	168
Great Western	113
Lejon	129
Noilly Pratt	136
Taylor	136

Vermouth, sweet
C&P	156
Gallo	150
Gancia	185
Great Western	172
Lejon	174
Noilly Pratt	172
Taylor	175

Cordials and Liqueurs, 1 oz

Amaretto	80
Anise	82
Anisette	
Bols	111
DuBouchett	85
DeKuyper	95
Garnier	82
Mr. Boston	90
Mr. Boston Connoisseur	64

1

Apricot
   Bols   96
   Dolfi   100
   DuBouchett   65

B & B   94

Benai   110

Benedictine   110

Blackberry
   Bols   90
   Dolfi   89
   DuBouchett   68

Brandy, flavored
   Bols   100
   DuBouchett   87
   Garnier   6
   Leroux   90
   Mr. Boston   100
   Mr. Boston Connoisseur   75

Cherry liqueur
   Bols   96
   DeKuyper   75
   Dolfi   87
   DuBouchett   72
   Hiram Walker   82
   Leroux   82

Chocolate
   Vandermint   90

Claristine
   Leroux   114

Coffee
Tia Maria   92
Pasha   100
Crème de almond
DuBouchett   100
Crème de apricot
Mr. Boston   90
Mr. Boston Connoisseur   65
Crème de banana
Garnier   90
Mr. Boston   90
Mr. Boston Connoisseur   65
Crème de cacao
Bols   100
Dolfi   100
DuBouchett   100
Garnier   100
Hiram Walker   100
Mr. Boston   90
Mr. Boston Connoisseur   65
Crème de cassis
Leroux   87
Mr. Boston   90
Crème de menthe   100
Crème de noisette   90
Crème de noyaux
Bols   115
Mr. Boston   99
Crème de peach
Mr. Boston Connoisseur   65

1

Curaçao	100
Drambuie	110
Grenadine	81
Kirsch	80
Kümmel	
DuBouchett	
48 proof	65
70 proof	83
Garnier	75
Hiram Walker	71
Leroux	75
Mr. Boston	78
Lochon Ora	
Leroux	89
Peach Liqueur	
Bols	96
DeKuyper	82
Dolfi	103
DuBouchett	67
Hiram Walker	81
Leroux	85
Raspberry Liqueur	
Dolfi	80
DuBouchett	56
Rock & Rye	
DuBouchett	
60 proof	78
70 proof	86
Garnier	83
Mr. Boston	90

1

Mr. Boston Connoisseur	65

Schnapps, peppermint

DuBouchett	85
Garnier	83
Hiram Walker	78
Leroux	87
Mr. Boston	77

Sloe Gin

Bols	85
DeKuyper	70
Dolfi	114
DuBouchett	70
Garnier	83
Mr. Boston	67

Triple Sec

Bols	104
Dolfi	107
DuBouchett	61
Garnier	83
Hiram Walker	105
Leroux	104
Mr. Boston	100

BEER, ALE, MALT LIQUOR,
12 oz

Andeker	160
Black Horse Ale	162
Brauhaus	150

1

Buckeye	144
Budweiser	156
Budweiser Malt Liquor	160
Busch Bavarian	155
Carling Black Label	160
Carlsberg Light	159
Carlsberg Dark	240
Champale Malt Liquor	157
Country Club Malt Liquor	163
Coors	138
Eastside Lager	145
Falstaff	150
Gablinger's	99
Goebel	145
Grand Union	150
Grenzquell	150
Hamms	138
Heidelberg	133
Heidelberg Light	129
Heileman's	158
Kingsbury	146
Knickerbocker	160
Meister Brau	144
Meister Brau Draft	144
Meister Brau Lite	96
Michelob	160
Michelob Light	134
Miller	150
Miller Lite	96
Natural Light	110

1

Old Dutch	150
Old Milwaukee	144
Old Ranger	150
Pabst Blue Ribbon	150
Pabst Light	100
Pabst Extra Light	70
Pearl	145
Pilser's	152
Red Cap Ale	159
Rheingold	160
Schaefer	158
Schlitz	148
Schlitz Light	96
Schmidt's	142
Stag	151
Stroh Bohemian	136
Stroh Bock	155
Stroh Light	115
Tuborg USA	140
Tudor	150

Near Beer, 12 oz

Goetz Pale	78
Kingsbury	45

1

Nonalcoholic Beer, 12 oz

Maltcrest	70
Metbrew	70
Zing	65

SOFT DRINKS, 8 oz

Note: Virtually all sodas that are called *low calorie,* *sugar free,* or *dietetic* contain 2 calories or less.

Aspen	105
Birch Beer	
Canada Dry	110
Pennsylvania Dutch	109
Yukon Club	116
Bitter lemon	
Canada Dry	104
Schweppes	128
Bitter orange	
Schweppes	124
Bubble Up	97
Cactus Cooler	120
Cherry	
Cott	123
Crush	121

Fanta	117
Mission	122
Club soda, all brands	0
Coconut	
Yoo-Hoo	117
Coffee	
Hoffman	88
Cola	
Canada Dry	110
Coca-Cola	96
Pepsi-Cola	104
Royal Crown	109
Pepsi Light	47
Shasta	90
Cream	
Canada Dry	127
Fanta	130
Shasta	90
Schweppes	115
Dr. Brown's Cel-Ray Tonic	89
Dr. Nehi	98
Dr. Pepper	98
Fruit punch	
Shasta	110
Fruit mix	
Wyler's	88
Ginger Ale	
Canada Dry	85
Fanta	85
Nehi	91

1

1

Crush	120
Fanta	114
Hi-C	101
Nedick's	121
Nehi	124
Patio	128
Schweppes	118
Shasta	114
Sunkist	125
Pineapple	
Canada Dry	`110
Purple Passion	
Canada Dry	120
Quinine Water	
Canada Dry	95
Fanta	84
Schweppes	88
Rondo	
Schweppes	100
Root Beer	
A&W	114
Berks County	116
Canada Dry Barrelhead	110
Canada Dry Rooti	110
Dad's	105
Fanta	103
Hires	100
On Tap	105
Patio	110
Royal Crown	113

Schweppes	105
Shasta	100
7-Up	97
Sprite	95
Squirt	91
Strawberry	
Canada Dry	120
Crush	121
Fanta	121
Nehi	116
Shasta	94
Yoo-Hoo	124
Sun-Drop	118
Teem	93
Tahitian Treat	
Canada Dry	130
Tiki	100
Tonic	
Canada Dry	90
Schweppes	88
Shasta	66
Upper 10	101
Vanilla	
Yoo-Hoo	125
Vanilla Cream	
Canada Dry	130
Wild Cherry	
Canada Dry	130
Wink	120

COFFEE AND TEA, 6 oz

Coffee	
regular	2
instant	4
flavored	
General Foods	
Cafe Francais	60
Cafe Vienna	60
Orange Cappuccino	60
Suisse Mocha	60
Postum	10
Tea, bags or loose	1
Tea, bottled or canned	
Lipton	84
sugar free	1
No-Cal	0
Tea, instant	
Lipton lemon-flavored	3
100% Tea	0
Nestea	1
Tender Leaf	1
Tea, mix, iced, lemon-flavored	
Our Own (A&P)	62
Lipton	40
Nestea	15
with sugar	70

Salada	57
Wyler's	56

FRUIT AND VEGETABLE JUICES, 6 oz

Fresh

Grapefruit	70
Lemon or Lime	45
Lemon or Lime, 1 Tbsp	3
Orange	
California	85
Florida	80
Valencia	85
Peach Nectar	90
Tangerine	80

Bottled and Canned

Apple	
Ann Page	90
Heinz	75

Beverages

Musselman's	80
Mott's	80
Pillsbury	60
Seneca	80
Welch's	90

Apple-Cranberry

Lincoln	104

Apricot nectar

Del Monte	100
Heart's Delight	194
Heinz	104
Libby's	110
Seneca	75

Cranberry-Apple

Cranapple	120

Fig

Real Fig	135

Fig and Prune

Fig 'n' Prune	135

Grape

Heinz	120
Seneca	110
Welch's	120

Grapefruit

Del Monte	70
Heinz	70
Libby's	75
Ocean Spray	70
Seneca	55
Stokely-Van Camp	60

1

Welch's	75
Grapefruit-Orange	
Seneca	77
Grenadine syrup, nonalcoholic, 1 oz.	
Garnier	100
Giroux	104
Lemon, 1 Tbsp	
ReaLemon	4
Rose's	5
Lime, 1 Tbsp	
ReaLime	6
Orange	
Del Monte	80
Heinz	75
Libby's	90
Welch's	90
Orange-Grapefruit	
Del Monte	80
Libby's	80
Stokely-Van Camp	70
Peach Nectar	
Del Monte	100
Libby's	90
Heart's Delight	89
Pear Nectar	
Del Monte	110
Libby's	100
Heart's Delight	95
Pineapple	
Del Monte	100

Dole	93
Heinz	95
Seneca	68
Stokely-Van Camp	110

Pineapple-Grapefruit

Del Monte	90

Pineapple-Orange

Ann Page	87
Del Monte	90
Hi-C	94
Lincoln	97

Prune

Ann Page	140
Del Monte	120
Heinz	130
Mott's	140
RealPrune	130
Seneca	130
Sunsweet	124
Welch's	150

Tomato

Campbell's	35
Del Monte	35
Heinz	38
Hunt's	43
Libby's	39
Sacramento	32
Seneca	27
Stokely-Van Camp	33
Townhouse	35

Welch's	38
Vegetable	
Campbell V-8	35
Vegemato	32

Frozen Juice

Grape	
Minute Maid	99
Snow Crop	99
Grapefruit	
Bird's Eye	68
Minute Maid	75
Snow Crop	75
Lemon	
Minute Maid	40
Orange	
Bright and Early	90
Minute Maid	90
Snow Crop	120
Stokely-Van Camp	90
Orange-Grapefruit	
Bird's Eye	72
Minute Maid	76
Pineapple	
Dole	101
Minute Maid	92

Pineapple-orange
Minute Maid	94
Dole	77

Tangerine
Minute Maid	86
Snow Crop	85

Dairy-Packed Juice, 8 oz

Grapefruit
Tropicana	75

Orange
Borden	96
Kraft	90
Sealtest	96
Tropicana	83

Orange-Grapefruit
Kraft	90

Orange-Pineapple
Ann Page	87
Hi-C	94
Kraft	96

FRUIT-FLAVORED DRINKS, ALL TYPES, 6 oz

Apple
  Ann Page — 90
  Hi-C — 90
Apple-Grape
  Mott's — 90
  Welch's — 92
Apricot-Apple
  BC — 92
Cherry
  Ann Page — 90
  Hi-C — 75
Citrus Cooler
  Ann Page — 90
  Hi-C — 90
Cranberry
  Ann Page — 120
  Ocean Spray — 105
  Seneca — 120
  Welch's — 105
Cranberry-Apple
  Ann Page — 135
  Lincoln — 103
  Mott's — 95
  Ocean Spray — 135

Cranberry-Apricot
Ocean Spray 105

Cranberry-Grape
Ocean Spray 105
Welch's 120

Cranberry-Orange
Knox 59

Cranberry-Prune
Ocean Spray 120

Grape
Ann Page 90
Hi-C 90
Welch's 90

Grape-Apple
BC 107

Grapefruit
Ann Page 80
Sealtest 90
Tropicana 70

Lemon
Sealtest 90

Lemonade
Bird's Eye 74
Borden 78
Country Time 67
Hi-C 75
Minute Maid 75
ReaLemon 76
Sealtest 80
Snow Crop 75

Stokely-Van Camp	80
Wyler's	67
Lemon-Limeade	
Minute Maid	75
Snow Crop	75
Limeade	
Bird's Eye	75
Minute Maid	75
Snow Crop	75
Orange	
A&P	80
Ann Page	90
Bird's Eye	105
Borden	85
Hi-C	125
Minute Maid	125
Start	120
Stokely-Van Camp	114
Tang	120
Tropicana	93
Welch's	135
Orange-Pineapple	
Ann Page	120
BC	120
Start	120
Peach	
Hi-C	120
Pineapple-Grapefruit	
Dole	120

Punch
- *Ann Page*   120
- *Hawaiian Punch*   120
- *Hi-C*   130
- *Mott's*   120
- *Stokely-Van Camp*   114
- *Tropicana*   93
- *Welch's*   130
- *Wyler's*   85

Raspberry
- *Wyler's*   85

Strawberry
- *Hi-C*   120
- *Wyler's*   85

Tangerine
- *Hi-C*   120

Wild Berry
- *Ann Page*   120
- *Hi-C*   115

CHAPTER 2

Dairy

BUTTER AND MARGARINE

Butter
½ cup (¼ lb)	815
1 Tbsp	100

Butter, whipped
½ cup	540
1 Tbsp	65

Margarine, 1 Tbsp

Imitation
Mazola	50
Parkay	50
Weight Watchers	50

Regular and Soft, all brands	100
Diet, all brands	50
Spread	
Blue Bonnet	80
Fleishmann	80
Parkay	70
Whipped, all brands	70

CHEESE, 1 oz unless noted

American	
Borden	104
Kraft	90
Blue	
Borden	105
Casino	100
Kraft	99
Brie	
Dorman	100
Kraft	100
Camembert	
Borden	85
Kraft	85
Caraway	
Kraft	111
Cheddar	
Borden	113
Kraft	113

Colby
Borden   111
Kraft   111

Cottage, 1 cup
creamed
  Borden   240
  Breakstone   230
  Breakstone low-fat   180
  Foremost   212
  Friendship   360
  Kraft   214
  Lucerne   240
  Meadow Gold   134
  Sealtest   114

partly creamed
  Meadow Gold   204
  Sealtest   176

uncreamed, potstyle
  Borden   196
  Breakstone   170
  Kraft   206
  Sealtest   180

low fat
  Borden   180
  Breakstone   180
  Friendship   200
  Lucerne   200
  Viva   200
  Weight Watchers   180

Cream cheese
Borden	96
Kraft Philadelphia Brand	98

Edam
Dorman	105
House of Gold	105

Farmer's
Breakstone	30
Dutch Garden	100
Friendship	38
Wispride	100

Fondue
Swiss Knight	60

Fontina
Kraft	114

Frankenmuth
Kraft	113

Gjetost
Kraft	135

Gorgonzola
Kraft	112

Gouda
Borden	86
Kraft	108

Gruyère
Borden	101
Kraft	108
Swiss Knight	101

Leyden
Kraft	80

Liederkranz
   Borden   86
Limburger
   Borden   97
   Dorman   100
   Kraft   98
   Mountain Valley   100
Monterey Jack
   Borden   103
   Casino   100
   Kraft   103
Mozzarella
   Borden   79
   Kraft   79
   Dorman   85
Muenster
   Borden   85
   Dorman   90
   Kraft   100
Neufchâtel
   Borden   73
   Kraft   69
Nuworld
   Kraft   104
Parmesan, grated, 1 Tbsp
   Buitoni   23
   Kraft   27
   La Rosa   33
   Lucerne   25

Parmesan & Romano, grated, 1 Tbsp
Borden   30
Kraft   30
Pimiento
Borden   104
Kraft   104
Port Salut
Dorman   100
Kraft   100
Premost
Kraft   134
Provolone
Borden   93
Kraft   99
Ricotta
Borden   42
Kraft   99
Romano, grated, 1 Tbsp
Buitoni   21
Kraft   26
Roquefort
Borden   107
Kraft   105
Sap Sago
Kraft   76
Sardo Romano
Kraft   110
Scamorze
Kraft   100

⎡2

Swiss
Borden 104
Dorman 90
Kraft 104
Sage
Kraft 113
Tilsit
Dorman 95

Cheese Food

American
Borden 92
Kraft 77
Blue
Borden 82
Borden Vera Blue 91
Wispride 100
Cheddar
Wispride 100
Jalapeno pepper
Kraft 93
Munst-ett
Kraft 101
Pimiento
Borden 91
Pauley Swiss 90
Velveeta 90
Pizza
Kraft 80

Sharp
 Kraft 93
Swiss
 Borden 91
 Kraft 91

Cheese Spread

American
 Borden 85
 Kraft 77
 Kraft Old English 97
American with Bacon
 Borden 80
 Kraft 92
Blue
 Borden 82
 Roka 80
 Wispride 92
Cheddar
 Snack Mate 85
 Wispride 97
Garlic
 Borden 82
 Kraft 86
Limburger
 Borden 82

Mohawk Valley	70
Moose	70
Pimiento	
Cheez Whiz	76
Kraft	77
Snack Mate	90
Smoked	
Borden	80
Velveeta	80

CREAM, 1 Tbsp

half and half	
Borden	19
Meadow Gold	27
Sealtest	20
light	
Borden	25
Foremost	30
Sealtest	35
medium	
Borden	41
Sealtest	42
heavy (whipping)	
Borden	52

Foremost	52
Lucerne	10
Sealtest	52

Sour Cream, 1 Tbsp

Borden	29
Borden half and half	29
Borden imitation	25
Foremost	30
Sealtest	29

Non-Dairy Creamers, 1 Tsp

coffee creamers
Carnation Coffee-Mate	11
Meadow Gold	9
Pet Cremora	11

whipped toppings
Reddi-Whip	7
Sta-Whip	8

EGGS

Chicken

raw, boiled, or poached

medium	72
large	82
extra large	94

raw, white only

medium	15
large	18
extra large	20
1 cup	125

raw, yolk only

medium	53
large	60
extra large	68

fried

medium	85
large	97
extra large	113

scrambled or omelet

medium	99
large	110
extra large	127

Duck, raw	130
Goose, raw	266
Turkey, raw	135

Egg Mixes, Commercial

Imitation
  Morningstar Farms Scramblers, ½ cup   130
  Tillie Lewis Eggstra, 1 pkt   101
  Fleishmann Egg Beaters, ½ cup   81
Omelets, 1 pkt
  Plain
    Durkee   604
    Durkee dry mix   112
  with bacon
    Durkee   620
    Durkee dry mix   125
  with cheese
    Durkee   617
    Durkee dry mix   127
    McCormick   130
    Schilling   128
  Western
    Durkee   604
    Durkee dry mix   112
    McCormick   115
    Schilling   115
Scrambled
  Durkee   124
  with bacon
    Durkee   180
  with sausage and potatoes
    Swanson   452

MILK, 8 oz

Buttermilk
Borden
.1% fat   88
.5% fat   90
1% fat   107
1.5% fat   110
2% fat   122
3% fat   158
Friendship 1.4% fat   120
Golden Nugget .8%   92
Light 'n Lively .8% fat   95
Lucerne 1.5% fat   120
Sealtest 2% fat   114

Skim
Borden .1% fat   81
Lucerne
0% fat   90
1% fat   110
2% fat   130
Meadow Gold
.5% fat   87
2% fat   130
Sealtest .1% fat   79

Skim Fortified
Borden   81
Borden Lite Line   117
Borden Hi Protein   132

Gail Borden	81
Light 'n Lively	114
Sealtest	137
Whole	
Borden	160
Foremost	154
Lucerne	160
Meadow Gold	166
Sealtest	150
Whole Fortified	
Gail Borden	159
Sealtest Multivitamin	151

Milk Beverages, 8 oz unless noted

Cherry-vanilla	
Borden	291
Chocolate	
Borden	210
Meadow Gold	190
Sealtest	175
Chocolate fudge	
Borden	284
Chocolate mixes	
Carnation Instant, 1 pkt	130
Carnation Slender, 1 pkt	110
Nestle's Quik	215

Ovaltine, 1 oz	105
Pillsbury, 1 pkt	295
Safeway, 2 tsp	215
Sealtest	195
Chocolate malt mix	
Carnation Instant, 1 pkt	130
Carnation Slender, 1 pkt	110
Eggnog, dairy packed	
Borden	
4.7% fat	260
6% fat	302
8% fat	375
Carnation, 1 pkt	130
Meadow Gold	327
Sealtest	324
Malt	
Borden	80
Carnation	90
Ovaltine	100
Mocha	
Borden	291
Strawberry	
Borden	287
Carnation, 1 pkt	130
Pillsbury, 1 pkt	290
Vanilla	
Borden	291
Carnation, 1 pkt	130

YOGURT, 8 oz

Plain
Borden Lite-Line	140
Borden Swiss Style	167
Breakstone	144
Dannon	150
Light 'n Lively	140
Lucerne	160
Pet	157
Viva	180

Flavored, all flavors
Borden	270
Breyer's	270
Dannon	210
Light 'n Lively	240
Meadow Gold	270
Viva	250

Frozen
Danny
In-A-Cup, 8 oz.	180
On-A-Stick, uncoated	65

CHAPTER 3

Breads, Crackers, Flour

BREAD, 1 slice, approximately 1 oz unless noted

Bran
  Brownberry   75
Corn & Molasses
  Pepperidge Farm   71
Cinnamon Raisin
  Thomas   60
Cracked Wheat
  Pepperidge Farm   66

Tasty Bake	70
Date Nut	
Thomas	100
French	
Pepperidge Farm	79
Wonder	75
Garlic	
Stouffer	80
Gluten	
Thomas	32
Hollywood	70
Honey Bran	
Pepperidge Farm	58
Honey Wheatberry	
Arnold	90
Pepperidge Farm	60
Italian	
Pepperidge Farm	81
Naturel	
Arnold	65
Nut	
Brownberry	85
Oatmeal	
Brownberry	82
Pepperidge Farm	66
Profile	52
Protein	
Thomas	45
Pumpernickel	
Arnold	75

Pepperidge Farm   79
Raisin
  Plain
    Arnold   75
    Thomas   66
  with cinnamon
    Brownberry   85
    Pepperidge Farm   75
    Thomas   65
  with nuts
    Brownberry   95
Rice Cakes
  Spiral   36
Rye
  Arnold   50
    Jewish   75
    soft   75
  Brownberry   65
  Pepperidge Farm   82
  Tasty Bake   91
  Wonder   75
Sourdough
  Di Carlo   71
Wheat
  Arnold
    Granary   71
    Branola   90
    Brick Oven   60
    Melba Thin   40
  Brownberry   85

Buckwheat	75
Colonial	72
Home Pride	75
Pepperidge Farm	70
Pepperidge Farm Very Thin	40
Thomas	50
Wonder	75
Wheat Germ	
Pepperidge Farm	69
White	
Arnold	
Brick Oven, .8 oz slice	65
Brick Oven, 1.1 oz slice	85
Country	95
Hearthstone Country	70
Melba Thin	40
Brownberry Sandwich	75
Brownberry Thin	70
Butternut	75
Colonial	75
Daffodil Farm	58
Fresh Horizons	50
Hart	75
Heartstone	85
Home Pride	75
Homestyle	75
Manor	75
Pepperidge Farm	75
Pepperidge Farm Sandwich	72
Sweetheart	75

Tasty Bake	72
Thomas	64
Weight Watchers	35
Wonder	75
Whole Wheat	
Pepperidge Farm	61
Thomas	65

Bread, Canned, ½ inch slice

Banana Nut	
Dromedary	71
Brown	
B&M	52
Chocolate Nut	
Cross & Blackwell	65
Dromedary	87
Date Nut	
Dromedary	75
Fruit and Nut	
Cross & Blackwell	77
Orange Nut	
Cross & Blackwell	76
Dromedary	78
Spice Nut	
Cross & Blackwell	65

Bread Mixes

White, ¼ loaf	
Pillsbury	460
Cornbread, 1 pkg	
Pillsbury	320
Aunt Jemima	330

BISCUITS, MUFFINS AND ROLLS

Biscuits, Baking Powder, 1 biscuit

1869 Brand	105
prebaked	100
Pillsbury	70
Tenderflake	60

Biscuits, refrigerated, 1 biscuit

Plain

Ballard	50
Borden	59
Hungry Jack	95
Flaky	90

Pillsbury	55
Flaky Baking Powder	67
Tenderflake	
Baking Powder	60
Buttermilk	
Hungry Jack	
Extra Rich	65
Flaky	80
Fluffy	100
Pillsbury	50
Big Country	95
Extra Light	55
Tenderflake	55
Corn Bread	
Pillsbury	95

Muffins, frozen, 1 muffin

Blueberry	
Thomas	110
Howard Johnson	121
Morton	120
Rounds	110
Pepperidge Farm	130
Corn	
Howard Johnson	118
Morton	
regular	130

Rounds	125
Pepperidge Farm	140
Thomas	120
English	
Thomas	130
Orange	
Howard Johnson	115
Raisin Bran	
Pepperidge Farm	130

Muffins, Mix, 1 muffin

Apple Cinnamon	
Betty Crocker	160
Banana Nut	
Betty Crocker	185
Blueberry	
Betty Crocker	120
Corn	
Betty Crocker	160
Orange	
Betty Crocker	155
Pineapple	
Betty Crocker	125

Muffins, packaged

Bran
Thomas 118
Cinnamon Raisin
Pepperidge Farm 140
Corn
Thomas 180
Toast-r-Cakes 120
English
Di Carlo 145
Hostess 145
Thomas 140
Wonder 144
Honey Butter
Arnold Orowheat 150
Onion
Thomas 130
Raisin
Wonder 155
Sourdough
Wonder 130
Wheat
Home Pride 140

3

Muffins, refrigerated, 1 muffin

Apple Cinnamon
Pillsbury   155
Corn
Pillsbury   130

Rolls, 1 roll

Hard Rolls
Pepperidge Farm   120
   French, 3 oz   264
   French, 5 oz   395
   Hearth   64
   Sesame Crisp   76
Wonder   82
Sandwich and Hamburger Rolls
Arnold
   Dutch Egg Buns   130
   Francisco   180
   Soft   110
   Hamburger   110
   Hot Dog   110
Colonial   160
Pepperidge Farm   120
Wonder   160
Soft Rolls
Arnold

Deli-Twist	110
Finger, 24's and 12's	55
Francisco	100
Refrigerator	95
Ballard	95
Borden	
Gem Flake	70
Onion	95
Colonial	80
Home Pride	90
Pepperidge Farm	
Butter Crescent	130
Dinner	65
Finger	60
Golden Twist	120
Old Fashioned	37
Parkerhouse	60
Party	35
Pillsbury	
Butterflake	110
Crescent	95
Hot Roll Mix	95
Wonder	
Buttermilk	85
Pan	105
Sweet Rolls, refrigerated	
Caramel	
Pillsbury	160
Cinnamon	
Ballard	100

Hungry Jack	145
Pillsbury	114
Orange	
Pillsbury	130
Scones	
Hostess	188

CRACKERS, 1 piece

Bacon Flavored
Keebler	15
Nabisco Bacon Thins	11

Barbecue
Chit Chat	14
Sunshine	17

Butter
Hi-Ho	17
Keebler	
Butter Thins	17
Club	15
Townhouse	19
Nabisco	15
Ritz	17
Tam-Tams	13

Butter-cheese
Ritz	18

3

Caraway
Caraway Crazy 15
Cheese
Cheese-Nips 5
Cheese Tid-Bits 4
Cheez-It 6
Che-Zo 5
Keebler 11
Pepperidge Farm 12
Cheese-peanut Butter
Keebler 14
Chicken
Chicken In a Biskit 10
Club
Keebler 15
Flings Curls
Nabisco 10
Gold Fish
Pepperidge Farm, 1 oz 140
Ham
Nabisco 12
Hi-Ho
Sunshine 18
Kavli Flatbread 35
Matzos
Goodman's Square 110
Goodman's Tea 75
Horowitz-Margareten 130
Manischewitz
Egg 132

Egg 'N Onion	113
Regular	110
Tam Tams	14
Tasteas	115
Thin Tea	110
Whole Wheat	122

Onion
Keebler	15
Manischewitz	13
Nabisco	13
French Onion	12
Pepperidge Farm	12

Potato
Chippers	14
Potato Piffles	17

Ritz
Nabisco	17

Rye
Keebler Rye Toast	18
Peek Frean	30
Ry Krisp	24

Saltines
Jacob's	
Biscuits for Cheese	35
English Cream	110
Keebler	
Salt-Free	15
Saltines	14
Sea Toast	60
Whole Wheat Sea Toast	58

Nabisco
   Premium   12
   Royal Lunch   54
   Uneeda   22
Sunshine   11

Sesame
   Keebler   16
   Meal Mates   22
   Sesame Sillys   15
   Sunshine   24

Shapies   10

Sip'N Chips   10

Sociables
   Nabisco   10

Toasts
   Dutch Rusk   60
   Holland Rusk   39
   Keebler   15
   Old London   11
   Pepperidge Farm   11
   Sunshine All-Rye   21

Soda and water crackers
   Huntley & Palmer   35
   Jacob's Golden Puffs   34
   Keebler Milk Lunch   27
   Waldorf   18
   Zesta   14

Tomato-onion
   Sunshine   15

3

Town House
 Keebler   15
Triangle Thins
 Nabisco   8
Twig?
 Nabisco   14
Waffle crackers   22
Waverly wafers
 Nabisco   18
Wheat
 Nabisco
  Wheat Toast   15
  Wheat Thins   9
Zwieback
 Nabisco   31

OTHER BREAD PRODUCTS

Breadcrumbs, 1 cup   450

Contadina   450
4C plain   410
4C seasoned   400

Breadsticks, 1 piece

onion
Stella D'Oro   35
plain
Stella D'Oro   40
sesame
Stella D'Oro   38
dietetic
Stella D'Oro   43

Croutons, ½ cup unless noted

bacon
Bel Air   80
Brownberry   90
cheese and garlic
Bel Air   100
garlic
Bel Air   80
Italian cheese
Bel Air   100
plain
Bel Air   60
seasoned
Bel Air   90
Brownberry   90

Stuffing, mixes, 1 pkg

Pepperidge Farm	110
Stove Top	170
Uncle Ben's	120

FLOURS, 1 cup

Buckwheat	
dark	325
light	340
Cake	370
Carob	250
Corn	485
Corn Starch, 1 Tbsp	35
Lima Bean	430
Peanut	225
Rye	
light	315
medium	310
dark	420
Soybean, defatted	325
full fat	300
low fat	310
Tortilla	
corn	410

3

wheat	450
Wheat, all purpose	485
bread	500
cake	430
gluten	530
self-rising	440
whole wheat	400
White	400
Unbleached	400

Meal, 1 cup

Almond	696
Corn	433
Cracker	450
Graham cracker	465
Matzo	444

CHAPTER 4

Cereal, Pancakes, Waffles and French Toast

CEREAL, ready to eat, 1 cup

bran

All-Bran, *Kellogg's*	190
40% Bran Flakes, *Kellogg's*	140
100% Bran Flakes, *Nabisco*	150
40% Bran Flakes, *Post*	125
Bran Chex, *Ralston Purina*	165
Bran & Prune Flakes, *Post*	120
Bran & Raisin Flakes, *General Mills*	125
Raisin Bran, *Kellogg's*	200
Raisin Bran, *Ralston Purina*	200
Raisin Bran, *Safeway*	200

Raisin Bran with Sugar Coating, *Post*	178
Bran-Buds with wheat germ, *Kellogg's*	200

corn

Country Corn Flakes, *General Mills*	80
Kix, *General Mills*	75
Corn Flakes, *Kellogg's*	110
Toasties Corn Flakes, *Post*	110
Corn Chex, *Ralston Purina*	110
Corn Flakes, *Ralston Purina*	110
Corn Flakes, *Safeway*	110
Corn Flakes & Blueberries, *Post*	110
Corn Flakes & Strawberries, *Post*	110
Sugar Frosted Flakes, *Kellogg's*	144
Sugar Pops, *Kellogg's*	105
Honeycomb Corn, *Post*	85
Sugar Sparkled Flakes, *Post*	149
Cocoa Puffs, *General Mills*	110
Trix, *General Mills*	111

corn and oats

Sugar Sparkled Twinkies, *General Mills*	112
Cap'n Crunch, *Quaker*	163
Crisp, *Quaker*	105

oats

Cheerios, *General Mills*	110
OK's, *Kellogg's*	83
Alpha-Bits, *Post*	110
Crispy Critters, *Post*	110
Fortified Oat Flakes, *Post*	165
Life, *Quaker*	160
Lucky Charms, *General Mills*	110

Frosty O's, *General Mills*	110
Sugar Jets, *General Mills*	111
Stars, *Kellogg's*	112
Fruit Loops, *Kellogg's*	112

rice

Rice Krispies, *Kellogg's*	105
Puffed Rice, *Quaker*	45
Crispy Rice, *Ralston Purina*	110
Rice Chex, *Ralston*	110
Crispy Rice, *Safeway*	110
Puffa Puffa Rice, *Kellogg's*	120
Rice Honeys, *Nabisco*	150
Rice Krinkles, *Post*	127
Cocoa Crispies, *Kellogg's*	113

wheat

Buc Wheats, *General Mills*	146
Total, *General Mills*	110
Wheat Stax, *General Mills*	81
Wheaties, *General Mills*	108
Crumbles, *Kellogg's*	140
Pep, *Kellogg's*	106
Shredded Wheat, *Kellogg's* 1 biscuit	63
Shredded Wheat, *Nabisco* 1 biscuit	92
Grape Nuts Flakes, *Post*	150
Puffed Wheat, *Quaker*	38
Shredded Wheat, *Quaker* 1 biscuit	68
Wheat Chex, *Ralston Purina*	165
Sugar Crisp, *Kellogg's*	147
Sugar Smacks, *Kellogg's*	110
Wheat Honeys, *Nabisco*	153

4

mixed grains

Concentrate, *Kellogg's*	310
Product 19, *Kellogg's*	106
Special K, *Kellogg's*	70
Apple Jacks, *Kellogg's*	112
Team Flakes, *Nabisco*	83
Grape Nuts, *Post*	400
Quake, *Quaker*	118

Cereal, cooked, 1 cup

barley

Quaker	172

corn meal mush

Quaker	128

farina

Cream of Wheat

Instant	133
Mix'N Eat	140
Quick	133
Regular	133
H-O	168
Pillsbury	120
Quaker	100

grits

Quaker

Instant	79

Instant with cheese flavor, 1 pkt	105
Instant with imitation bacon, 1 pkt	100
Instant with imitation ham, 1 pkt	100
3-Minute Brand, ¼ cup	150

oats

H-O	150
Quaker	160

oatmeal

Quaker	143

rice

Cream of Rice	145

rye

Con Agra	360

whole wheat

Quaker Pettilohns	145

PANCAKES, FRENCH TOAST, WAFFLES AND OTHER BREAKFASTS, 1 piece unless noted

Breakfast Bars, frozen

Carnation	210
General Mills	190

4

Crepes, mix, 6″ crepe
Aunt Jemima — 55
French Toast, frozen
Aunt Jemima — 85
  with cinnamon — 100
Downyflake — 135
Swanson, with sausage, 1 pkg — 335
French Toast, mix
McCormick — 119
Fritters, frozen
Mrs. Paul's — 120
Pancakes, frozen
Downyflake — 75
Swanson, with sausage, 1 pkg — 500
Pancakes, frozen batter
Aunt Jemima — 70
Pancakes, mix, 4″ pancake
Aunt Jemima
  Easy Pour — 60
  buckwheat — 80
  buttermilk — 70
Betty Crocker — 70
Hungry Jack — 75
  blueberry — 112
  buttermilk — 80
  Extra Lights — 60
Pancake-Waffle, mix
Aunt Jemima — 70
  buttermilk — 100
  whole wheat — 80

Log Cabin	60
buttermilk	75
Waffle, mix	
Aunt Jemima	100
Downyflake	60
Jumbo	89

CHAPTER 5

Beans, Pasta and Rice

BARLEY, 1 cup

pearled, light	698
pearled, Pot or Scotch	696

BEANS DRIED,
1 cup unless noted

Broadbeans, raw, immature seeds, 8 oz	238
Broadbeans, raw, mature seeds, 8 oz	768

Black, dry, uncooked, 8 oz	768
Chick peas	
8 oz	817
1 cup	720
Great Northern	212
Lima, immature seeds	190
Lima, mature seeds, dried	262
Mung, dried	714
Pea or Navy, dried	224
Pinto (red Mexican), uncooked	663
Red Kidney	220
White, dried	224

Baked Beans, ½ cup

B & M	180
Campbell	148
barbecue	171
with franks	181
with pork	147
Heinz	140
Campside	180
with franks	184
with pork	150
Howard Johnson's	163
Morton House	160

PASTA, 1 cup unless noted

Dry

egg noodles

Goodman's	175
La Rosa	190
La Rosa spinach	200
Pennsylvania Dutch	200
Prince	190
Ronzoni	200

macaroni

Goodman's	170
La Rosa	180
Prince	170
Ronzoni	175

spaghetti

Buitoni	175
Goodman's	160
La Rosa	165
Prince	160
Ronzoni	165

5

Macaroni, canned, bagged, frozen and mixes

with beef

Banquet	260
Chef Boy-Ar-Dee	235
Franco-American	220
Green Giant Boil-in-Bag, 1 pkg	240
Morton	260
Stouffer's, 1 pkg	380

with beef and cheese

Banquet	300
Green Giant Boil-in-Bag, 1 pkg	330
Hormel, 7½ oz can	340
Howard Johnson's	330
Morton	215
Mac-A-Roni & Cheddar	290
Pennsylvania Dutch	310
Stouffer's, 1 pkg	520
Swanson	200

with cheese sauce

Franco-American	225
Heinz	230
MacaroniO's	180
Noodle-Roni	290
Scallop-A-Roni	275

with chili sauce

Fiesta Mac-A-Roni	270

creole style

Heinz, 8¾-oz can	169

Noodles, canned, frozen and mixes

Almondine
Betty Crocker, 1 pkg   960
with beef
Heinz, 8½ oz can   170
with beef in gravy
College Inn   238
with beef in tomato sauce
College Inn   238
with beef
Hormel, 7½-oz can   240
with beef sauce
Pennsylvania Dutch   260
Betty Crocker   170
with butter sauce
Pennsylvania Dutch   300
with cheese
Noodle-Roni   650
with cheese sauce
Pennsylvania Dutch   300
with cheese sauce and sour cream
Noodle-Roni Romanoff   362
with chicken
Dinty Moore, 7½-oz can   215
with chicken sauce
Noodle-Roni   250
Pennsylvania Dutch   300
Twist-A-Roni   250

5

Romanoff

Betty Crocker, 1 pkg	800
Stouffer's, 1 pkg	500

Stroganoff

Betty Crocker, 1 pkg	900
Pennsylvania Dutch	630

with tuna

Stouffer's, 1 pkg	400

Noodles, Italian style, canned, frozen and mixes

Cannelloni, 8 oz

Weight Watchers	275

Eggplant Parmigiana, 8 oz

Buitoni	421
Weight Watchers	172

Lasagna, 8 oz unless noted

Buitoni	250
with meat sauce	340
Chef Boy-Ar-Dee	
canned	241
mix	265
Golden Grain, 1 pkg	720
Green Giant	
Boil-in-Bag, 1 pkg	310
Oven Bake, 1 pkg	300
Hormel	
7½-oz can	270
10-oz can	370

Lean Cuisine, 11 oz	260
Lean Line, 10 oz	270
Roman	274
Stouffer's, 1 pkg	385
Swanson, 1 pkg	540
Weight Watchers	215

Manicotti, 8 oz
Buitoni	395
with sauce	350
Lean Line	270

Ravioli, 8 oz
Buitoni	
cheese	575
meat	680
Chef Boy-Ar-Dee	
cheese	263
meat	210
Franco-American, 7½-oz can	220
La Rosa	
cheese	205
meat	218
Roman	
cheese	496
meat	552

Ravioli Parmigiana, 8 oz
Buitoni	
cheese	301
meat	381

5

Rotini
Franco-American, 7½-oz can	200
with meatballs	230

Shells
Buitoni, 8 oz	235
Lean Line, 11 oz	270

Spaghetti, all with tomato sauce, 1 cup unless noted
Banquet with meatballs	212
Betty Crocker, 1 pkg	170
Buitoni	
with meatballs	250
with mushrooms	170
Chef Boy-Ar-Dee	
with cheese sauce	180
with meat	260
with meat sauce	250
with meatballs	250
with mushrooms	225
Franco-American	
with cheese sauce	200
with meat	290
with meatballs	260
Spaghetti-Os	
with cheese	200
with meatballs	228
Golden Grain	275
Green Giant, Boil-in-Bag	
with meatballs	280

Heinz
with cheese sauce	175
with franks	310
with meat sauce	173

Hormel
with meat	280
with meat sauce	205

Kraft	260
La Rosa with meatballs	230
Lean Cuisine	280
Libby's with meatballs	95
Morton, frozen, 1 pkg	220
Stouffer's, 1 pkg	445
Swanson, 1 pkg	290

Ziti
Buitoni, 8 oz	270
Lean Line, 10 oz	270
Weight Watchers, 1 pkg	350

RICE, 1 cup unless noted

Plain
Ann Page, whole pkg	1000
Bird's Eye	260
Carolina	200

5

Green Giant	230
Minute	300
Rice-A-Roni, whole pkg	780
River	200
Uncle Ben's	200
Uncle Ben's, brown	250

Flavored

beef
   Uncle Ben's — 210

beef and cracked rice
   Betty Crocker — 416

beef and vermicelli
   Minute — 300
   Rice-A-Roni — 315

beef and cheese sauce
   Betty Crocker — 350

chicken
   Uncle Ben's — 210

chicken with crumb topping
   Betty Crocker — 365

chicken and vermicelli
   Minute — 300
   Rice-A-Roni — 321

curry
   Uncle Ben's — 205

fried Chinese and vermicelli
   Rice-A-Roni — 375

ham and vermicelli
   Rice-A-Roni — 300

pilaf
  Uncle Ben's   290
Frozen
  Green Giant   160
   Medley   220
   Pilaf   240
   Verdi   140
Spanish, canned
  Heinz   190
  La Rosa   155
  Libby's   57
  Stokely-Van Camp   180

Bulgur (parboiled wheat), 1 cup

Club Wheat, dry   630
Hard Red Winter Wheat, dry   605
  canned, unseasoned   225
  seasoned   246
White Wheat, dry   555

CHAPTER 6

Soup

CANNED OR FROZEN,
1 cup unless noted

with bacon
  Ann Page 140
  Campbell's 174
  Town House 155
with hot dogs
  Campbell's 168
with smoked pork
  Heinz 160

Bean, black
  Campbell's 95
  Crosse & Blackwell 118

Bean, lima
  Manischewitz 93

Beef
plain
  Campbell's 105
  Lipton 200
with barley
  Manischewitz 83
  Wyler's 72
with cabbage
  Manischewitz 62
with low sodium
  Campbell's, 7¼-oz can 170
mushroom
  Lipton 45
with noodles
  Campbell's 69
  Heinz 74
  Manischewitz 65

Lipton	67
Souptime, 1 envelope	30
Town House	75
Wyler's	50
with vegetables	
Manischewitz	61
Borscht	
Manischewitz	72
Rokeach	75
Bouillon, 1 cube	
beef	
Herb-Ox	6
Knorr-Swiss	15
Maggi	6
Wyler's	7
chicken	
Herb-Ox	6
Knorr-Swiss	17
Maggi	7
Wyler's	8
onion	
Herb-Ox	10
Wyler's	8
vegetable	
Herb-Ox	6
Wyler's	6
Bouillon, instant, 1 tsp	
beef	
Maggi	6
Wyler's	10

chicken
  Maggi   7
  Wyler's   6
Broth
beef
  Campbell's   26
  College Inn   15
  Swanson, 6¾-oz can   25
  Weight Watchers, 1 pkt   10
chicken
  Campbell's   43
  College Inn   32
  Richardson & Robbins   17
  Swanson, 6¼-oz can   25
chicken with noodles
  College Inn   45
chicken with rice
  College Inn   45
  Richardson & Robbins   45
Celery, cream of
  Ann Page   60
  Campbell's   160
  Heinz   180
  Town House   100
Cheddar cheese
  Campbell's   150
Chickarina
  Progresso   100
Chicken
  Lipton   220

Chicken alphabet
  Campbell's   88
Chicken with barley
  Manischewitz   83
Chicken, cream of
  Ann Page   90
  Lipton   106
  Souptime, 1 pkt   100
  Town House   95
Chicken with dumplings
  Campbell's   100
Chicken gumbo
  Campbell's   59
Chicken with kasha
  Manischewitz   41
Chicken with low sodium
  Campbell's, 7½-oz can   170
Chicken noodle
  A & P   67
  Ann Page   70
  Campbell's   66
  Golden Grain   74
  Heinz   35
  Lipton   54
  Manischewitz   46
  Souptime, 1 pkt   30
  Town House   75
  Wyler's   44
Chicken with rice
  Ann Page   50

6

6

Mushroom
Plain

Campbell's	80
Golden Grain	95
Souptime	80
Wyler's	151

with barley

Manischewitz	72

bisque

Crosse & Blackwell	127

cream of

Ann Page	120
Campbell's	217
Heinz	200
Knorr-Swiss	116
Lipton	92
Town House	124
Wyler's	151

Noodle

Lipton	50

with chicken broth

Ann Page, 1 pkt	225
Lipton	60

with ground beef

Campbell's	98

Onion

Ann Page, 1 pkt	125
Crosse & Blackwell	57
Golden Grain	33

Knorr-Swiss	45
Lipton	35
Souptime, 1 pkt	20
Wyler's	146
Onion with mushroom	
Lipton	35
Oriental style	
Lipton	210
Oyster stew	
Campbell's	
canned	146
frozen	196
Pea	
green	
Campbell's	148
Golden Grain	73
Knorr-Swiss	71
Lipton	136
Souptime low sodium, 1 pkt	70
with ham	
Campbell's	130
low sodium, 7½-oz can	150
split	
Manischewitz	133
split with ham	
Ann Page	180
Campbell's	180
Heinz	150
Town House	154

Pepper pot
    Campbell's   105
Petite Marmite
    Crosse & Blackwell   41
Potato
  Plain
    Lipton   100
  cream of
    Campbell's   190
  with leek
    Wyler's   155
Schav
    Manischewitz   11
    Rokeach   12
Scotch broth
    Campbell's   90
Senegalese
    Crosse & Blackwell   75
Shrimp, cream of
    Crosse & Blackwell   113
    Campbell's   230
Sirloin burger
    Campbell's   177
Steak and potato
    Campbell's   160
Stockpot
  vegetable
    Lipton   220
  vegetable-beef
    Campbell's   96

Tomato
Ann Page	80
Campbell's	84
Heinz	87
Lipton	93
Manischewitz	61
Progresso	110
Souptime, 1 pkt	70
Town House	87

Tomato bisque
Campbell's	126

Tomato
low sodium
Campbell's 7¼-oz can	130

with rice
Ann Page	90
Campbell's	106
Manischewitz	78

with vegetables
Golden Grain	86
Lipton	69

Tuna Creole
Crosse & Blackwell	70

Turkey
Plain
Campbell's	138

with noodles
Ann Page	75

Heinz	83
Lipton	74
Town House	83
low sodium	
Campbell's, 7¼-oz can	60
with vegetables	
Ann Page	60
Campbell's	78
Vegetable	
Plain	
Ann Page	70
Campbell's	83
Old Fashioned	74
Lipton	70
Italian	100
Knorr-Swiss	56
Manischewitz	63
Town House	83
Wyler's	81
with beef	
Ann Page	80
Campbell's	81
low sodium, 7¼-oz can	80
Old Fashioned	79
Heinz	66
Lipton	53
Town House	66
cream of	
Souptime, 1 pkt	80

Soup 6

CHAPTER 7

Meat, Poultry and Seafood

MEAT, FRESH

Retail cuts of meat are frequently weighed with bone first, *then* they are trimmed, cooked and weighed for their yield. So for instance 1 lb. of pork loin chops are weighed raw with bone, but after they are trimmed and cooked, their yield is 5.9 oz.

7

Beef, choice-grade, retail cuts

Chuck, arm, roast, or steak; boneless, lean with fat
raw, 1 lb   1,012
  braised, drained
    10.7 oz (yield from 1 lb)   879
    4 oz   328
    1 cup, chopped   405
    1 cup, ground   318

Chuck, arm, roast, or steak, lean only
  braised, drained
    9.1 oz (yield from 1 lb)   498
    4 oz   219
    1 cup, chopped   270
    1 cup, diced   212

Chuck, rib roast or steak, lean with fat
raw, 1 lb   1,597
  braised, drained
    10.7 oz (yield from 1 lb)   1,298
    4 oz   484
    1 cup, chopped   598
    1 cup, ground   470

Chuck, stewing; boneless, lean with fat
raw, 1 lb   1,166
  stewed, drained
    10.7 oz (yield from 1 lb)   994
    4 oz   371
    1 cup, chopped   458

Chuck, stewing; boneless, lean only
raw, 1 lb   717

stewed, drained

10.7 oz (yield from 1 lb)	651
4 oz	243
1 cup, chopped	300

Club steak, 16% bone, lean with fat

raw, 1 lb	1,443

broiled

9.8 oz (yield from 1 lb raw)	1,262
4 oz without bone	515

Club steak, 16% bone, lean only

broiled

5.7 oz (yield from 1 lb)	393
4 oz without bone	277

Flank steak, boneless, lean only

raw, 1 lb	653

braised, drained

10.7 oz (yield from 1 lb)	596
4 oz	222

Ground, lean with 10% fat

raw, 1 lb	812
broiled, 12 oz (yield from 1 lb)	745

Ground, lean with 21% fat

raw, 1 lb	1,216
broiled, 11.5 oz (yield from 1 lb)	932

Plate, boneless, lean with fat

raw, 1 lb	1,216

simmered, drained

10.7 oz (yield from 1 lb)	1,313
4 oz	490

Plate, boneless, lean only
  simmered, drained
    6.5 oz (yield from 1 lb)   368
    4 oz   226
Porterhouse steak, 9% bone, lean with fat
  raw, 1 lb   1,603
  broiled
    10.6 oz (yield from 1 lb)   1,400
    4 oz without bone   527
Porterhouse steak, 9% bone, lean only
  broiled
    6.1 oz (yield from 1 lb)   385
    4 oz without bone   254
Rib roast, boneless, lean with fat
  raw, 1 lb   1,819
  roasted
    11.7 oz (yield from 1 lb)   1,456
    4 oz   499
    1 cup, chopped   616
    1 cup, ground   484
Rib roast, boneless, lean only
  roasted
    7.5 oz (yield from 1 lb)   511
    4 oz   273
    1 cup, chopped   337
    1 cup, ground   265
Round steak, boneless, lean with fat
  raw, 1 lb   894
  braised or broiled
    11.1 oz (yield from 1 lb)   820

4 oz   296

Round steak, boneless, lean only
braised or broiled
    9.5 oz (yield from 1 lb)   507
    4 oz   296

Rump roast, boneless, lean with fat
raw, 1 lb   1,374
roasted
    11.7 oz (yield from 1 lb)   1,149
    4 oz   394
    1 cup, chopped   486
    1 cup, ground   382

Rump roast, boneless, lean only
roasted
    8.8 oz (yield from 1 lb)   516
    4 oz   236
    1 cup, chopped   291
    1 cup, ground   229

Sirloin steak, double bone, 18% bone, lean with fat
raw, 1 lb   1,240
broiled
    9.6 oz (yield from 1 lb)   1,110
    4 oz without bone   463

Sirloin steak, double bone, 18% bone, lean only
broiled
    6.3 oz (yield from 1 lb)   372
    4 oz without bone   272

Sirloin steak, round-bone, 7% bone, lean with fat
raw, 1 lb   1,316

broiled

10.9 oz (yield from 1 lb)	1,192
4 oz without bone	439

Sirloin steak, round-bone, 7% bone, lean only
broiled

7.2 oz (yield from 1 lb)	420
4 oz without bone	235

T-bone steak, 11% bone, lean with fat

raw, 1 lb	1,596

broiled

10.4 oz (yield from 1 lb)	1,395
4 oz without bone	537

T-bone steak, 11% bone, lean only
broiled

5.8 oz (yield from 1 lb)	368
4 oz without bone	253

Beef, prepared and specialty cuts

Beef, corned

raw, 1 lb	1,596

cooked

10.7 oz (yield from 1 lb)	1,131
4 oz	422

Beef, dried, creamed, home recipe

8 oz	350

Beef, hearts, lean only
raw

8 oz	245

braised	
4 oz	213
1 cup, chopped	273
Beef, kidneys	
raw, 8 oz	294
braised	
4 oz	286
1 cup, chunks	353
Beef, liver	
raw, 1 lb	635
fried, 4 oz	260
Beef pancreas, raw, 4 oz	
fat	358
medium fat	321
lean	160
Beef suet, raw, 1 oz	242
Beef sweetbreads (thymus)	
yearlings, raw, 1 lb	939
yearlings, braised, 4 oz	365
Beef, tongue	
very fat, raw, trimmed, 8 oz	615
fat, raw, trimmed, 8 oz	524
medium-fat, raw, trimmed	
8 oz	470
braised, 4 oz	277
Beef, tripe, 4 oz	
commercial	113
pickled	70

7

Lamb, fresh

Leg, lean with fat
  raw, with bone, 1 lb   845
  roasted, with bone
    9.4 oz (yield from 1 lb)   745
  raw, boneless, 1 lb   1,007
  roasted, boneless
    11.2 oz (yield from 1 lb)   887
    4 oz   317
    1 cup, chopped   391
Leg, lean
  roasted, with bone
    7.8 oz (yield from 1 lb with fat)   411
  roasted, boneless
    9.7 oz (yield from 1 lb with fat)   491
    4 oz   211
    1 cup, chopped   260
Loin chops, with bone, lean with fat
  raw, 1 lb   1,146
  broiled
    10.1 oz (yield from 1 lb)   1,023
    4 oz   407
    1 chop, 3.4 oz   341
    1 chop, 2.5 oz   255
Loin chops, with bone, lean only
  broiled
    6.9 oz (yield from 1 lb)   368
    4 oz   213
    1 chop, 2.3 oz   122

1 chop, 1.7 oz	92
Rib chops with bone, lean with fat	
raw, 1 lb	1,229
broiled	
9.5 oz (yield from 1 lb)	1,091
4 oz	462
1 chop, 3.1 oz	362
1 chop, 2.4 oz	273
Rib chops with bone, lean only	
broiled	
6 oz (yield from 1 lb)	361
4 oz	239
1 chop, 2 oz	120
1 chop, 1.5 oz	91
Shoulder, lean with fat	
raw with bone, 1 lb	1,082
roasted, with bone	
9.5 oz (yield from 1 lb)	913
raw, boneless, 1 lb	1,275
roasted, boneless	
11.2 oz (yield from 1 lb)	1,075
4 oz	383
1 cup, chopped	473
Shoulder, lean only	
roasted, with bone	
7 oz (yield from 1 lb)	410
roasted, boneless	
8.3 oz (yield from 1 lb)	482
4 oz	233
1 cup, chopped	287

7

Lamb's quarters
raw, trimmed, 1 lb | 195
boiled, drained
    4 oz | 36
    1 cup | 64

Lamb hearts
raw, 8 oz | 368
braised
    4 oz | 295
    1 cup, chopped | 377

Lamb kidneys
raw, 8 oz | 238

Lamb liver
raw, 1 lb | 617
broiled, 4 oz | 296

Lamb tongue
raw, trimmed, 8 oz | 452
braised, 4 oz | 288

Lamb sweetbreads (thymus), 4 oz
raw | 106
braised | 200

Ham, retail cuts (see also Pork)

Boiled, 8 oz (about 8 slices) | 531
Fresh, lean with fat
raw, 1 lb with bone and skin | 1,188

baked
   9.2 oz (yield from 1 lb)   980
raw, 1 lb without bone and skin   1,397
baked
   10.9 oz (yield from 1 lb)   1,152
   4 oz   424
   1 cup, chopped   524
   1 cup, ground   411

Fresh, lean only
baked, with bone and skin
   6.8 oz (yield from 1 lb)   421
baked, without bone and skin
   8.1 oz (yield from 1 lb with fat)   495
   4 oz   246
   1 cup, chopped   304
   1 cup, ground   239

Light-cured, lean with fat
raw, with bone and skin, 1 lb   1,100
baked, with bone and skin
   11.3 oz (yield from 1 lb)   925
raw, without bone and skin, 1 lb 1,279
baked, without bone and skin
   13.1 oz (yield from 1 lb)   1,075
   4 oz   328
   1 cup, chopped   405
   1 cup, ground   318

Light-cured, lean only
baked, with bone and skin
   8.7 oz (yield from 1 lb with fat)   460

baked, without bone and skin
   10.2 oz (yield from 1 lb with fat)   539
baked, without bone and skin
   4 oz   328
   1 cup, chopped   405
   1 cup, ground   318
Long-cured, dry, unbaked
  medium-fat, lean with fat, with bone and skin,
   4 oz   384
  lean, lean with fat, with bone and skin, 4 oz 302
Ham, minced, 4 oz   259

Pork, fresh

Boston butt, shoulder, with bone and skin, lean with fat
  raw, 1 lb   1,220
  roasted, 10.2 oz (yield from 1 lb)   1,024
Boston butt, shoulder, without bone and skin, lean with fat
  raw, 1 lb   1,302
  roasted
   10.9 oz (yield from 1 lb)   1,087
   1 cup, chopped   494
   1 cup, ground   388
Boston butt, shoulder, with bone and skin, lean only
  roasted, 8.1 oz (yield from 1 lb with fat)   559

Boston butt, shoulder, without bone and skin, lean only
  roasted
    8.6 oz (yield from 1 lb with fat)   595
    1 cup, chopped   342
    1 cup, ground   268
Loin chops, with bone, lean with fat
  raw, 1 lb   1,065
  broiled
    8.2 oz (yield from 1 lb)   911
    1 chop, 2.7 oz   305
    1 chop, 2 oz   227
Loin chops without bone, lean with fat
  raw, 1 lb   1,352
  broiled
    10.4 oz (yield from 1 lb)   1,153
    4 oz   411
Loin chops, with bone, lean only
  broiled
    5.9 oz (yield from 1 lb with fat)   454
    1 chop, 2 oz   151
    1 chop, 1.5 oz   113
Loin chops, without bone, lean with fat
  raw, 1 lb   1,065
  baked or roasted, 8.6 oz (yield from 1 lb)   883
Loin roast, without bone, lean with fat
  raw, 1 lb   1,352
  baked or roasted
    10.9 oz (yield from 1 lb)   1,115
    4 oz   411
    1 cup, chopped   507

Loin roast, with bone, lean only
  baked or roasted
    6.9 oz (yield from 1 lb with fat)   495
    1 cup, chopped   356
Loin roast, without bone, lean only
  baked or roasted
    8.7 oz (yield from 1 lb with fat)   627
    4 oz   288
    1 cup, chopped   356
Picnic, shoulder, with bone and skin, lean with fat
  raw, 1 lb   1,083
  simmered, 8.4. oz (yield from 1 lb)   890
Picnic, shoulder, without bone and skin, lean with fat
  raw, 1 lb   1,315
  simmered
    10.2 oz (yield from 1 lb)   1,085
    4 oz   424
    1 cup, chopped   524
Picnic, shoulder, with bone and skin, lean only
  simmered, 6.2 oz (yield from 1 lb with fat)   373
Picnic, shoulder, without bone and skin, lean only
  simmered
    7.6 oz (yield from 1 lb with fat)   456
    4 oz   241
    1 cup, chopped   297
Spareribs, with bone, lean with fat
  raw, 1 lb   976
  braised
    6.3 oz (yield from 1 lb)   792
    4 oz   499

Pork, specialty cuts, hog

Hearts
raw, 4 oz	128
braised, 4 oz	221
braised, 1 cup	283

Kidneys, raw, 8 oz 240

Liver
raw, 1 lb	594
fried, 4 oz	205

Pancreas (Sweetbreads), 4 oz 274

Spleen, raw, 4 oz 122

Tongue, 4 oz
raw, trimmed	244
braised	287

Pork, specialty cuts, pig, 4 oz

Feet, pickled	227
Salt Pork	
with skin	1,137
without skin	888
Stomach, scalded	274

7

Pork, cured, retail shoulder cuts (for other cured cuts see Bacon and Ham)

Boston butt, with bone and skin, lean with fat
  unbaked, 1 lb   1,277
  baked or roasted, 11 oz (yield from 1 lb)   1,030
Boston butt, without bone and skin, lean with fat
  unbaked, 1 lb   1,320
  baked or roasted
    11.8 oz from 1 lb   1,109
    4 oz   374
    1 cup, chopped   462
    1 cup, ground   363
Boston butt, with bone and skin, lean only
  baked or roasted, 9.1 oz (yield from 1 lb with fat)   629
Boston butt without bone and skin, lean only
  baked or roasted
    9.8 oz (yield from 1 lb with fat)   678
    4 oz   276
    1 cup, chopped   340
    1 cup, ground   267
Picnic, with bone and skin, lean with fat
  unbaked, 1 lb   1,060
  baked or roasted, 9.7 oz (yield from 1 lb)   888
Picnic, without bone and skin, lean with fat
  unbaked, 1 lb   1,293
  baked or roasted
    11.8 oz (yield from 1 lb)   1,085
    4 oz   366
    1 cup, chopped   452

1 cup, ground	355
Picnic, with bone and skin, lean only	
baked or roasted, 6.8 oz (yield from 1 lb with fat)	405
Picnic, without bone and skin, lean only	
baked or roasted	
8.3 oz (yield from 1 lb with fat)	496
4 oz	239
1 cup, chopped	295
1 cup, ground	232
Bacon, Canadian	
uncooked, 1 lb	980
fried, drained	
12 oz (approx. yield from 1 lb)	921
4 oz	311
1 slice 3⅜″ wide	58
Bacon, cured	
raw, 1 lb	3,016
fried, drained	
5.1 oz (approx. yield from 1 lb)	860
1 thick slice	72
1 medium slice	43
1 thin slice	30

Veal, fresh, retail cuts

Chuck cuts and boneless for stew, lean with fat	
raw, with bone, 1 lb	628
stewed, with bone, 8.4 oz (yield from 1 lb)	564

raw, without bone, 1 lb	785
stewed, without bone	
10.6 oz (yield from 1 lb)	703
4 oz	267
1 cup, chopped	329
Loin cuts, lean with fat	
raw, with bone, 1 lb	681
braised, or broiled, with bone	
9.5 oz (yield from 1 lb)	629
raw, without bone, 1 lb	821
braised or broiled, without bone	
11.4 oz (yield from 1 lb)	758
4 oz	245
1 cup, chopped	328
Plate (breast of veal), lean with fat	
raw, with bone, 1 lb	828
braised or stewed, with bone,	
8.3 oz (yield from 1 lb)	718
raw, without bone, 1 lb	1,048
braised or stewed, without bone	
10.6 oz (yield from 1 lb)	906
4 oz	344
Rib roast, lean with fat	
raw, with bone, 1 lb	723
roasted, with bone, 8.5 oz (yield from 1 lb)	648
raw, without bone, 1 lb	939
roasted, without bone	
11 oz (yield from 1 lb)	842
4 oz	305
1 cup, chopped	377

    1 cup, ground   296

Round with rump (roasts and leg cutlets), lean with fat

    raw, with bone, 1 lb   573

    braised or broiled, with bone

        8.7 oz (yield from 1 lb)   534

    raw, without bone, 1 lb   744

    braised or broiled, without bone

        11.3 oz (yield from 1 lb)   693

        4 oz   245

        1 cup, chopped   302

Veal, specialty cuts

Calf hearts

    raw, 4 oz   140

    braised, 4 oz   236

      1 cup   302

Calf kidneys, raw, 8 oz   256

Calves' liver

    raw, 4 oz   212

    fried, 4 oz   296

Calf pancreas, 4 oz, raw   183

Calf tongue, 4 oz

    raw, trimmed   143

    braised   181

Calf sweetbreads (thymus), 4 oz

    raw   106

    braised   192

7

Cold Cuts, Sausages and other meats

Beaver, roasted, 8 oz.	563
Bockwurst	
1 lb (approx 7 links)	1,198
1 link (approx 2.3 oz)	172
Bologna	
without binders	
chub, 1 slice (3″ x ⅛″)	36
ring, 12 oz ring (15″ x 1⅜″)	942
sliced, 1 slice (approx 1 oz)	79
with cereal	
chub, 1 slice	34
ring, 12 oz ring	891
sliced, 1 slice	74
Brains, all types, fresh, raw, 8 oz	284
Capicola	
1 oz	141
1 slice	105
Cervelat, dry	
1 oz	128
4 slices	54
Frankfurter's without binders	
1 lb	1,343
1 frank (5″ x ¾″)	133
Frog's legs, raw	
whole, with bone, 1 lb	215
meat only, 4 oz	83
Meat Loaf, 4 oz	227

Muskrat, roasted, 4 oz	174
Rabbit, domesticated	
raw, whole, ready to cook, 1 lb	581
raw, meat only, 4 oz	184
stewed	
whole 8.6 oz (yield from 1 lb)	529
meat only	
4 oz	245
1 cup, chopped	302
1 cup, ground	238
Rabbit, wild	
whole, ready to cook, 1 lb	490
meat only, 4 oz	153
Raccoon, roasted, meat only, 4 oz	290
Reindeer, raw, lean meat only, 4 oz	144
Salami	
dry roll	
8¼ oz roll	1,053
1 slice	23
dry slice	
4 oz	509
1 slice	45
cooked	
8 oz	706
1 slice approx 1 oz	88
Sausage	
Blood pudding	
4 oz	447
1 slice	32

Polish
4 oz	345

pork, raw
2 oz patty	284
1 oz link (4" x ⅞")	141

pork, cooked
4 oz	543
1 patty	129
1 link	62

scrapple
4 oz	244
1 slice (⁹⁄₁₀ oz)	54

souse
4 oz	205
1 slice (1 oz)	51

Sheep tongue
raw, trimmed, 8 oz	602
braised, 4 oz	366

Snails, raw, 4 oz
meat only	103
Giant African, meat only	83

Spleen, all types, 4 oz — 125

Terrapin (diamondback), raw
in shell, 1 lb	106
meat only, 4 oz	126

Thuringer cervelat (summer sausage)
8 oz	697
1 slice (approx 1 oz)	87

Turtle, green, raw
in shell, 1 lb	97

meat only, 4 oz   101
Venison, raw, lean meat only, 4 oz   143

MEAT, COMMERCIALLY PACKAGED

Cured and processed meat, 1 oz unless noted

Bacon, cooked, 1 slice
  Hormel
    Black Label   35
    Range Label   45
    Red Label   37
  Oscar Mayer   40
  Swift   40
Bacon bits
  Wilson   140
Beef, chopped
  Eckrich, 1 slice   40
  Wilson   91
Beef, corned
  Dinty Moore   65
  Libby's   101
  Safeway   35

7

Beef, corned brisket
Swift   80
Wilson   45
Beef, dried
Swift   42
Beef, roast
Wilson   33
Beef, smoked
Safeway   35
  spicy   40
Beef steaks
Hormel   92
Bologna, 1 slice
Eckrich   90
  thick-sliced   160
Hormel   95
Swift   87
Wilson   87
Beef bologna
Eckrich   95
  Beef Smorgas   70
Oscar Mayer   70
Coarse ground bologna
Hormel   75
Fine ground bologna
Hormel   80
Garlic bologna
Eckrich   95
Braunschweiger
Oscar Mayer   100

Wilson   90

Frankfurters, 1 frank
  Eckrich   120
    Jumbo   190
    Skinless   150
  Hormel   180
    Wieners   105
  Oscar Mayer   140
  Wilson   140

Beef frankfurters, 1 frank
  Eckrich   150
    Jumbo   190
  Hormel
    Wieners   105
    Wranglers   160
  Oscar Mayer   140
  Vienna   130
  Wilson   136

Ham, lunch meat
  cooked
    Eckrich, 1 slice   40
    Hormel   35
    Safeway   50
    Oscar Mayer, 1 slice   30
  chopped
    Hormel   70
    Oscar Mayer, 1 slice   65
  chopped, smoked
    Eckrich   40

Ham, whole, canned, 1 oz
   Amber   110
   Oscar Mayer   32
   Swift   63
   Wilson
      boned and rolled   56
      fully cooked   48
      Tender Made   44

Ham, whole, packaged, 1 oz
   Hormel
      bone-in   52
      Cure 82   48
      Curemaster   35
   Oscar Mayer   36
   Swift   43
   Wilson   48

Ham steaks, 1 slice
   Oscar Mayer   70

Ham patties, 1 patty
   Hormel   200
   Swift   250

Ham and Cheese Loaf, 1 slice
   Oscar Mayer   75

Honey Loaf, 1 slice
   Eckrich   45
   Oscar Mayer   40

Liver, beef
   Swift   54

Liver cheese, 1 slice
   Oscar Mayer   110

Old Fashioned Loaf, 1 slice
  Eckrich   75
  Oscar Mayer   65
Olive Loaf, 1 slice
  Oscar Mayer   65
Pastrami, 1 slice
  Eckrich   47
  Safeway   40
Pepperoni
  Hormel   140
  Swift   150
Pickle Loaf, 1 slice
  Eckrich   85
  Oscar Mayer   65
Polish Sausage
  Eckrich   100
  Frito-Lay   73
  Hormel   80
Pork Butt
  Wilson   72
Pork Loin
  Eckrich   47
Pork Steaks
  Hormel   73
Salami
  Hormel   327
  Oscar Mayer, 1 slice   50
Sausage, beef
  Eckrich   95

Sausage, pork
Hormel 95
Wilson 135

Sausage links, 1 sausage
Hormel
  Brown 'n Serve 78
  Little Sizzlers 67
  Midget Links 112
Oscar Mayer 65
Swift 75

Sausage links, smoked, 1 sausage
Eckrich 190
  skinless 115
  Smok-Y-Links 75
Hormel 92
Oscar Mayer 140

Scrapple
Oscar Mayer 45

Sizzlean
Swift 50

Spam
Hormel 85

Summer Sausage
Swift 90

Thuringer
Hormel 100

Tripe
Libby's canned 35

Veal Steaks
  Hormel 35
    breaded 60
Vienna Sausage, 1 sausage
  Hormel 52
  Libby's 84
    with barbecue sauce 76

Canned Meat Entrees, 1 can, various sizes

Beef with barbecue sauce
  Morton House 240
Beef, corned with cabbage
  Hormel 150
Beef Goulash
  Hormel 240
Beef sliced with gravy
  Morton House 190
Chili con carne
  Hormel 340
  Libby's 130
  Morton House 340
Chili con carne with beans
  A&P 440
  Hormel 320
  Libby's 180
  Morton House 340
  Swanson 310
Hash, beef with potatoes
  Dinty Moore 270

Hash, corned beef

Ann Page	400
Armour Star	435
Bounty	405
Broadcast	480
Libby's	160
Morton House	480
Wilson	480

Hash, roast beef

Hormel	375

Meatballs in gravy

Chef Boy-Ar-Dee	315

Pork, sliced with gravy

Morton House	190

Salisbury Steak with mushroom gravy

Morton House	160

Sloppy Joe

Banquet	250
Gebhardt	280
Hormel	365
Libby's	
beef	163
pork	139

Stew, beef

Armour Star	200
B & M	163
Bounty	213
Dinty Moore	184
Heinz	253
Morton House	312

7

James River Smithfield	186
Libby's	78
Morton House	240
Swanson	190
Wilson	202

Stew, lamb
B & M	247

Stew, meatball
Chef Boy-Ar-Dee	218
Libby's	121
Morton House	290

Stew, Mulligan
Dinty Moore	240

Frozen Meat Entrees, 1 whole package, various sizes (see also pp 385-391, Frozen Dinners)

Beef
Banquet	
Cookin' Bag	124
Buffet Supper, 32 oz	782
Green Giant Boil-in-Bag	130
Seabrook Farms	263
Stouffer's	235
Swanson	190
Swanson Hungry-Man	330

7

Beef goulash
Seabrook Farms 198
Beef Pot Pie
Banquet 412
Swanson 443
Beef Stroganoff
Stouffer's 390
Green Pepper Steak
Stouffer's 350
Meat Loaf
Banquet
  Buffet Supper, 32 oz 1,445
  Cookin' Bag 224
  Man Pleaser 916
Morton 430
Swanson 330
Noodles and Beef
Banquet Buffet Supper, 32 oz 754
Salisbury Steak
Banquet 873
Green Giant Boil-in-Bag 390
Morton 490
Stouffer's 500
Swanson 370
Swanson Hungry-Man 640
Salisbury Steak with gravy
Banquet
  Buffet Supper, 32 oz 1,454
  Cookin' Bag 246

Green Giant Oven Bake	290
Sausage, cheese, and tomato pie	
Weight Watchers	390
Sloppy Joe	
Banquet Cookin' Bag	199
Green Giant Boil-in-Bag	160
Steak	
Weight Watchers	390
Stew, Beef	
Banquet Buffet Supper, 32 oz	700
Green Giant Boil-in-Bag	160
Lambrecht	432
Seabrook Farms	229
Stouffer's	310
Stuffed Cabbage with beef	
Green Giant Oven Bake	220
Stuffed Green Pepper with Beef	
Green Giant Oven Bake	200

Meat Substitutes, 1 piece or slice

Morningstar Farms	
Breakfast Links	62
Breakfast Patties	111
Breakfast Strips	38

7

Loma Linda

Bologna	190
Burgers	
Redi-Burger	150
Sizzle Burger	180
Frankfurters	110
Linketts	70
Little Links	45
Meatballs	48
Peanut Butter	
Nuteena	210
Proteena	160
Roast Beef	200
Salami	210
Sausage	
Breakfast Links	50
Breakfast Sausage	140
Swiss Steak	140
Tender Bits	20
Tender Rounds	50
Turkey	190
Vegeburger, 1 cup	240
Vegelona	160

POULTRY, FRESH

Chickens, fresh

Broilers
broiled, with skin, giblets	
7.1 oz (yield from 1 lb)	273
meat only, 4 oz	154

Capon, raw, ready to cook, 1 lb   382

Fryers
raw, ready to cook, 1 lb	382
fried, with skin, giblets	
8 oz (yield from 1 lb)	565
fried, without skin	
dark meat, 4 oz	249
light meat, 4 oz	223
1 back (approx 2 oz)	139
½ breast (approx 3.3 oz)	160
1 drumstick (approx 2 oz)	88
1 neck (approx 2 oz)	127
½ rib section (approx ¾ oz)	41
1 thigh (approx 2.3 oz)	122
1 wing (approx 1.8 oz)	82
skin only (approx 1 oz)	119

Roasters
raw, ready to cook, 1 lb	791
roasted, with skin, giblets	
8.4 oz (yield from 1 lb)	576

roasted, without skin, dark meat

4 oz	204
1 cup, chopped	258
1 cup, ground	202

roasted, without skin, light meat

4 oz	207
1 cup, chopped	255
1 cup, ground	200

Stewing hens or cocks

raw, ready to cook, 1 lb	987
stewed, with skin, giblets, 8 oz (yield from 1 lb)	708

stewed, without skin, dark meat

4 oz	235
1 cup, chopped	290
1 cup, ground	228

stewed, without skin, light meat

4 oz	204
1 cup, chopped	252
1 cup, ground	198

Chicken gizzards

raw, 1 lb	513

simmered

12 oz (yield from 1 lb)	497
4 oz	168
1 cup, chopped	215

Chicken hearts

raw, 4 oz	152

simmered

4 oz	221
1 cup, chopped	283

7

Chicken liver

raw, 1 lb	585
simmered	
4 oz	187
1 cup, chopped	231
1 liver 2" x 2" x ½"	45

Duck, fresh

Domesticated

raw, meat only, 4 oz	188
roasted, meat only, 4 oz	352

Wild

raw, meat only, 4 oz	157

Goose, fresh, domesticated

raw, whole, ready to cook, 1 lb	1,172
roasted	
whole, 8½ oz (yield from 1 lb)	1,022
meat only, 4 oz	266
meat and skin, 4 oz	503
Goose gizzards, raw, 1 lb	631
Goose liver, raw, 1 lb	826

7

Pheasant, fresh

raw, ready to cook, whole, 1 lb	596
raw, meat only, 4 oz	184

Quail, fresh, raw

whole, ready to cook, 1 lb	686
meat and skin only, 4 oz	196
giblets, 2 oz	100

Squab (Pigeon), fresh, raw

whole, dressed, 1 lb	569
meat only, 4 oz	162
light meat only, 4 oz	143

Turkey, fresh

raw, whole, ready to cook, 1 lb	722
roasted, whole, with giblets and skin 8.6 oz (yield from 1 lb)	644
roasted, dark meat without skin 4 oz	230

1 cup, chopped	284
1 cup, ground	223
roasted, light meat without skin	
4 oz	200
1 cup, chopped	246
1 cup, ground	194
roasted, skin only, 1 oz	256
giblets	
raw, 4 oz	170
simmered	
4 oz	254
1 cup, chopped	338
gizzards	
raw, 1 lb	712
simmered	
12 oz (yield from 1 lb)	659
4 oz	222
1 cup, chopped	284
hearts	
raw, 4 oz	169
simmered	
4 oz	245
1 cup, chopped	313
liver	
raw, 1 lb	626
simmered	
4 oz	197
1 cup, chopped	244

POULTRY, COMMERCIALLY CANNED, FROZEN, OR PACKAGED: 1 package, various sizes, unless noted (see also pp 385-391, Frozen Dinners)

Chicken

a la King

Banquet	138
Green Giant	170
Lambrecht	585
Stouffer's	330
Swanson	190

Boned

Hormel	110
Richardson & Robbins	328
Swanson	110

Chopped, 1 slice

Eckrich	47

Cacciatore

Seabrook Farms	248

Creamed

Stouffer's	300

Creole
  Weight Watchers 250
Croquette
  Howard Johnson's 505
Divan
  Stouffer's 335
and Dumplings
  Banquet 282
  Morton House, 8 oz 363
  Swanson 230
Escalloped
  Stouffer's 500
Fricasse, 1 cup
  College Inn 240
  Richardson & Robbins 229
Fried
  Banquet 259
  Morton 600
  Swanson 290
Livers with broccoli
  Weight Watchers 220
with Noodles
  Banquet 764
  Green Giant 250
  Howard Johnson 384
  Heinz 186
Pot Pie
  Banquet 412
  Morton 318
  Stouffer's 545

Swanson	430
Swanson Hungry-Man	770
with Rice	
Morton House, 8 oz	460
Smoked	
Safeway, 1 oz	50
Stew, 8 oz	
B & M	168
Bounty	221
Libby's	88
Swanson, 7½ oz	180
White meat with peas and onions	
Weight Watchers	270

Turkey

Boned	
Hormel	90
with Giblet gravy	
Banquet	128
Banquet Buffet Supper	170
Pot Pie	
Banquet	415
Morton	390
Stouffer's	460
Swanson	430
Swanson Hungry-Man	770

Slices
Banquet	98
Banquet Buffet Supper	564
Green Giant	100
Morton Country Table	390
Morton House canned	140
Swanson	260
Swanson Hungry-Man	380

Tetrazzini
Stouffer's	480

Smoked
Eckrich, 1 slice	47
Safeway, 1 oz	50

SEAFOOD, FRESH,
4 oz unless noted

Abalone, raw
in shell	47
meat only	111

Barracuda, Pacific, raw
meat only	129

Bass, black sea, raw
whole	41
meat only	106

Bass, all varieties, raw

whole	51
meat only	120

Blackfish, see Tautug

Bonito, raw

meat only	192

Butterfish, raw, meat only

gulf	108
northern	192

Catfish, raw, fillets | 117

Caviar, sturgeon

granular

1 oz	74
1 Tbsp	42

pressed

1 oz	90
1 Tbsp	54

Clams, raw, meat only

hard or round

1 pt	363
8 oz	182
4 cherrystones or 5 littlenecks	56

soft

1 pt	372
8 oz	186

Cod

raw, fillets, 8 oz	176

broiled, with butter

1 steak	352

7

4 oz	192
dehydrated, lightly salted	308
1 cup, shredded	158
dried, salted	148
Crab, steamed, 8 oz	
in shell	100
meat only	211
Crab, deviled	
8 oz	427
Crab, Imperial	
8 oz	334
Crayfish, raw	
in shell	10
meat only	82
Croaker, Atlantic	
raw, meat only	109
Croaker, white	
raw, meat only	95
Croaker, yellow	
raw, meat only	101
Cusk	
raw, meat only	85
steamed, meat only	120
Eulachon, see Smelt	
Finnan Haddie	
meat only	117
Flounder, fillets	
raw	89
baked with butter	229

155

Grouper, raw

whole	42
meat only	99

Haddock

raw

whole, 1 lb	172
fillets, 1 lb	360
fried, breaded, 4 oz	187

Halibut, Atlantic or Pacific

raw

whole, 1 lb	268
fillets, 1 lb	452
broiled with butter, fillets, 4 oz	199

Herring

Atlantic, raw

whole, 1 lb	405
meat only, 4 oz	200

Pacific

raw, meat only, 4 oz	111
salted (in brine), 4 oz	247
smoked, 4 oz	
bloaters	222
hard	340
kippers	239

Inconnu, raw

whole	104
meat only	166

Kingfish, raw

whole	52

meat only	119
Lake Herring (Cisco), raw	
whole	55
meat only	110
Lake Trout, raw	
whole	70
meat only	190
Ling Cod, raw	
whole	44
meat only	96
Lobster, northern	
in shell, 1 lb	
raw	107
cooked	112
Mackerel, Atlantic	
raw, 1 lb	
whole	468
fillets	866
broiled with butter, fillets,	
13 oz yield from 1 lb	861
4 oz	268
Mackerel, Pacific, raw	
whole	130
meat only	181
Mackerel, salted	345
Mackerel, smoked	248
Mullet, raw	
whole	88
meat only	166

Muskellunge, raw
  whole 60
  meat only 124
Mussels, Atlantic or Pacific, raw
  in shell 38
  meat only 108
Ocean Perch, Atlantic
  raw
    whole 31
    meat only 100
  fried, breaded 258
Ocean Perch, Pacific, raw
  whole 29
  meat only 108
Octopus, raw 83
Oysters, raw
  Eastern
    in shell, 1 lb 30
    meat only, 4 oz 75
    1 medium 20
  Pacific Western
    meat only, 4 oz 105
    1 medium 55
Oysters, cooked
  fried, breaded, 1 medium 25
Pickerel, raw 95
Perch, raw
  white
    whole 48
    meat only 134

yellow
whole	40
meat only	103

Pike, raw

blue
whole	45
meat only	100

northern
whole	26
meat only	100

walleye
whole	60
meat only	105

Pompano, raw
whole	106
meat only	188

Porgy, raw ... 52
meat only	127

Rockfish
raw	110
steamed	115

Roe, raw
carp, cod, haddock, herring, pike, and shad	148
salmon, sturgeon, and turbot	236

Sablefish, raw
whole	90
meat only	216

Salmon, raw

Atlantic
whole	160

meat only	246
King (Chinook) meat only	252
Salmon, smoked	200
Sand Dab, raw	
meat only	89
Sardines, Pacific	
raw, meat only	180
Sauger, raw	
whole	34
meat only	95
Scallops, meat only	
raw	92
steamed	127
Sea Bass, white	
raw, meat only	109
Shad, raw	
whole	92
meat only	192
Sheepshead, Atlantic, raw	
whole	60
meat only	128
Shrimp	
raw, whole	
in shell	72
shelled	100
fried, breaded	250
Skate	
raw, meat only	111
Smelt, raw	
whole	60

7

meat only	110
Snapper, Red and Gray, raw	
whole	55
meat only	106
Sole, raw	
whole	29
meat only (fillet)	90
Spanish Mackerel, raw	
whole	142
meat only	200
Spot	
raw, meat only	250
Squid	
raw, meat only	95
Sturgeon, meat only	
raw	105
steamed	180
Sturgeon, smoked	170
Sucker, carp	
raw	48
meat only	125
Sucker, white and mullet, raw	
whole	195
meat only	118
Swordfish, meat only	
raw	138
broiled in butter	185
Tautug (Blackfish), raw	
whole	37
meat only	101

7

Tilefish
  raw
    whole   46
    meat only   90
  baked, meat only   155
Tomcod, raw
  whole   34
  meat only   88
Trout, Brook, raw
  whole   56
  meat only   115
Trout, Rainbow, raw
  meat only   220
Tuna, raw, meat only
  bluefin   165
  yellowfin   150
Turbot, Greenland, raw
  whole   86
  meat only   166
Weakfish
  raw
    whole   66
    meat only   138
  broiled in butter   230
Whitefish, raw
  whole   82
  meat only   177
  smoked   177
Wreckfish
  raw, meat only   130

Yellowtail
raw, meat only   157

SEAFOOD, CANNED
AND FROZEN

Catfish, ocean
Gorton's, 1 pkg   286
Clams
Doxsee
6 oz   84
8 oz   112
12 oz   147
Howard Johnson's
5 oz   395
Croquettes, 1 pkg   608
Mrs. Paul's 1 cake   180
Thins, 1 cake   155
Sticks, 1 stick   48
Sau-Sea, 1 jar   99
Snow's   60
Cod, 1 pkg
fillets
Gorton's   355
San Juan   336
Ship Ahoy   336

sticks
Bird's Eye	552
Gorton's	830

Crab
Gold Seal, 1 can	185
Icy Point, 1 can	215
Mrs. Paul's, 1 cake	60
Pillar Rock, 1 can	216
Ship Ahoy, 8 oz	210
Wakefield's, 6 oz	160

Crepes, 5½ oz
Mrs. Paul's
Clam	280
Crab	240
Scallop	220
Shrimp	250

Croquettes
Howard Johnson's
Shrimp with Newburg Sauce	480

Eel, smoked
	185
Vita	402

Fish Au Gratin
Mrs. Paul's 1 pkg	250

Fish cakes, fillets and sticks, 1 piece
Mrs. Paul's	105
Beach Haven	110
Thins	160

Fish and Chips
Swanson, 1 pkg	290

Fish Parmesan
  Mrs. Paul's, 1 pkg   220
Flounder
  Mrs. Paul's, 1 pkg   110
  Weight Watchers, 1 pkg   160
Gelfilte Fish, 1 oz
  Manischewitz   23
  Mother's   14
  Rokeach   19
Haddock au Gratin
  Howard Johnson's   315
Haddock fillets
  Gorton's, 1 pkg   360
  Mrs. Paul's, 1 piece   115
Haddock with stuffing
  Weight Watchers, 1 pkg   180
Herring, pickled, 1 oz
  Vita   40
Oysters, 1 cup
  Bumblebee   172
Perch, fried, 1 piece
  Mrs. Paul's   125
Perch, ocean with broccoli
  Weight Watchers, 1 pkg   190
Salmon, canned, 1 can
  blueback
    Icy Point
      3¾-oz can   181
      7¾-oz can   376

Coho steak
  Icy Point
    3¾-oz can   162
pink
  Del Monte
    7¾-oz can   310
red
  Icy Point
    1-lb. can   775
  Pillar Rock
    3¾-oz can   181
    7¾-oz can   376
red sockeye
  Del Monte
    7¾-oz can   340
  Bumblebee
    1 cup   286
Sardines, 1 oz
  Del Monte   44
  Underwood
    in mustard sauce   52
    in soya bean oil   62
    in tomato sauce   330
Scallops
  Mrs. Paul's, 3½ oz   210
Seafood combination
  Mrs. Paul's   510
Shrimp
  Bumblebee, 1 can   90

Icy Point, 1 can	148
Pillar Rock, 1 can	148
Mrs. Paul's, 1 oz	57
Sau-Sea, 1 oz	80
Shad Roe	
Bumblebee, 1 can	259
Shrimp and Scallops	
Stouffer's, 1 pkg	400
Sole	
Mrs. Paul's, 4½ oz	160
Ship Ahoy, 1 pkg	310
with peas, mushrooms, and lobster sauce	
Weight Watchers, 1 pkg	200
Tuna, canned in oil, drained	
Bumblebee, 1 cup	334
Chicken of the Sea	
3¼-oz can	224
6½-oz can	447
9¼-oz can	636
12½-oz can	860
Del Monte, 6½-oz can	450
Gold Seal, 5-oz can	278
Icy Point, 5-oz can	278
Pillar Rock, 5-oz can	278
Snow Mist, 5-oz can	278
Van Camp, 6¼-oz can	440
Tuna, canned, solid, in water	
Bumblebee, 1 cup	300
Chicken of the Sea, 7-oz can	216

Tuna, creamed, with peas
  Green Giant Boil-in-Bag   140
Tuna Pot Pies
  Banquet   478
  Morton   385
  Star Kist   397
Turbot with peas and carrots
  Weight Watchers, 1 pkg   280

CHAPTER 8

Fruits and Vegetables

FRESH FRUITS AND VEGETABLES

Acerolas (West Indian Cherries)
whole, 1 lb	104
pitted, 4 oz	32
3 cherries	7

Amaranth
whole, 1 lb	100
leaves only, 1 lb	160

Apples
with skin	
1 lb	242

1 apple (3¼", 2 per lb)	123
1 apple (2¾", 3 per lb)	80
1 apple (2½", 4 per lb)	61
chopped, 1 cup	73
pared	
1 apple (3¼", 2 per lb)	107
1 apple (2¾", 3 per lb)	70
1 apple (2½", 4 per lb)	53
chopped, 1 cup	68
Apples, dehydrated	
uncooked	
8 oz	800
1 cup	355
cooked, sweetened	
8 oz	175
1 cup	195
Apples, dried	
uncooked	
8 oz	625
1 cup	234
cooked, unsweetened	
8 oz	177
1 cup	199
cooked, sweetened	
8 oz	254
1 cup	314
Apricots	
whole	
1 lb	217
1 apricot	18

    pitted, halves
       1 lb ... 231
       1 cup ... 79

Apricots, dehydrated
    uncooked
       8 oz ... 755
       1 cup ... 330
    cooked, sweetened
       8 oz ... 271
       1 cup ... 339

Apricots, dried
    uncooked
       8 oz ... 590
       1 cup ... 340
       10 medium halves ... 90
    cooked, unsweetened, with liquid
       8 oz ... 195
       1 cup ... 210
    cooked, sweetened, 1 cup ... 329

Artichokes
    raw, whole, 1 lb ... 85
    boiled, drained, 1 whole bud ... 67

Asparagus
    raw
       whole, 1 lb ... 66
       cuts, 1 cup ... 35
    boiled, drained
       1 medium spear ... 3
       cuts, 1 cup ... 29

8

Avocados, California

whole, 1 lb	589
peeled and pitted, 1 average	370
diced, 1 cup	260
mashed, 1 cup	390

Avocados, Florida

whole, 1 lb	389
peeled and pitted, 1 average	200
diced, 1 cup	190
mashed, 1 cup	300

Bamboo shoots, raw

8 oz	61
1 cup, cuts	40

Bananas

whole

1 large (10″)	119
1 medium (9″)	103
1 small (8″)	83

1 cup

sliced	135
mashed	190

Bananas, dehydrated

flakes, 1 cup	340

Bananas, red

whole, 1 average (7¼″)	118
sliced, 1 cup	135

Bean Sprouts, mung

uncooked

8 oz	80
1 cup	37

boiled, drained
8 oz	65
1 cup	35

Bean sprouts, soy
uncooked
8 oz	105
1 cup	48

boiled, drained
8 oz	86
1 cup	48

Beet greens
raw, trimmed, 1 lb	61

boiled, drained
8 oz	41
1 cup	26

Beets
raw, trimmed
1 lb	137
whole, 1 beet (2″)	21
diced, 1 cup	58

boiled, drained
whole, 1 beet	16
diced, 1 cup	58
sliced, 1 cup	66

Blackberries
1 lb	250
1 cup	84

Blueberries
1 lb	260
1 cup	90

Broccoli

raw

whole, 1 lb	90
trimmed, 1 lb	145

boiled, drained

8 oz	59
1 average stalk 6½ oz	47
cuts, 1 cup	40

Brussel Sprouts

raw

whole, 1 lb	200
trimmed, 1 lb	190

boiled, drained

8 oz	82
1 cup	55
1 average sprout	7

Cabbage, Chinese (Celery Cabbage), raw

whole, 1 lb	62
trimmed, 1 lb	65
cuts, 1 cup	11
strips, 1 cup	8

Cabbage, green

raw

whole, 1 lb	98
trimmed, 1 lb	110
chopped, 1 cup	22
sliced, 1 cup	17
ground, 1 cup	36
boiled, drained, 1 cup	30

Cabbage, dehydrated, 1 oz   87

Cabbage, red, raw
whole, 1 lb	127
trimmed, 1 lb	141
sliced, 1 cup	22

Cabbage, savoy, raw
whole, 1 lb	98
trimmed, 1 lb	109
sliced, 1 cup	17

Cabbage, spoon (Bakchoy)
raw	
whole, 1 lb	73
trimmed, 1 lb	70
cuts, 1 cup	11
boiled, drained, cuts, 1 cup	24

Cantaloupe
one 5-inch melon	95
cubed, 1 cup	48

Carambola, raw
whole, 1 lb	150
peeled and seeded, 8 oz	80

Carissas (Natal plums), raw
whole, 1 lb	273
peeled and seeded, 8 oz	155
sliced, 1 cup	105

Carrot
raw	
whole, 1 lb	156
whole scraped	
8 oz	95
1 medium	21

diced, 1 cup	60
slices, 1 cup	53
boiled, drained, 1 cup	45
Carrot, dehydrated, 1 oz	100
Casaba melon	
whole	61
cubed, 1 cup	45
Cauliflower	
raw	
whole, 1 lb	48
flowerets	
1 lb	120
1 cup	27
chopped, 1 cup	30
boiled, drained, 1 cup	29
Celeriac root, raw	
whole, 1 lb	155
pared, 1 root approx 1 oz	11
Celery	
raw	
whole, 1 lb	58
1 large outer stalk (8″)	7
1 small inner stalk (5″)	3
chopped, 1 cup	20
boiled, drained, 1 cup	22
Chard, Swiss	
raw	
whole, 1 lb	113
1 lb, then trimmed	104

boiled, drained
    leaves and stalks, 1 cup   26
    leaves only, 1 cup   32

Chayote
raw, 1 medium squash   56

Cherimoya, raw
whole, 1 lb   247
peeled and seeded, 8 oz   215

Cherries
sour, red
  whole
    1 lb   213
    1 cup   60
  pitted, 1 cup   90
sweet
  whole
    1 lb   286
    1 cup   82
  pitted
    1 cup   102
    1 average cherry   5

Chervil
raw, 1 oz   16

Chives, raw
whole, 1 lb   128
chopped, 1 Tbsp   1

Coconut, raw
in shell, 1 coconut (4½″ and 27 oz)   1,375
shelled, meat only, 4 oz   392

shredded, 1 cup
loosely packed 277
firmly packed 450

Coconut, dried, shredded
unsweetened
4 oz 750
1 cup 622
sweetened
4 oz 622
1 cup 515

Collards
raw
whole, 1 lb 180
leaves only, 1 lb 205
boiled
leaves only 60
with stems, 1 cup 43

Corn, sweet
raw, on the cob, 1 lb 240
boiled, drained
on the cob, 1 ear (5″) 70
kernels, 1 cup 140

Corn Salad, raw
whole, 1 lb 90
trimmed, 1 lb 95

Crab apples, raw
whole, 1 lb 280
trimmed 309

Cranberries
whole, 1 lb 200

without stems, 1 cup	52
chopped, 1 cup	50
Cranberries, dehydrated, 1 oz	100
Cucumber	
1 lb	65
1 average (7½″)	35
sliced, 1 cup	15
Currants	
black	
whole, 1 lb	240
trimmed, 1 cup	60
red or white	
whole, 1 lb	220
trimmed, 1 cup	55
Dandelion greens	
raw, trimmed, 1 lb	205
boiled, drained, 1 cup	
loosely packed	35
firmly packed	70
Dates, domestic	
whole, 1 lb	1,081
pitted, 1 lb	1,243
chopped, 1 cup	488
1 average date	22
Dock (Sorrel)	
raw, whole, 1 lb	89
boiled, drained, 1 cup	38
Eggplant	
raw	
whole, 1 lb	92

diced, 1 cup	50
boiled, drained, 1 cup	38˙
Elderberries	
whole, 1 lb	310
without stems, 8 oz	160
Endive (French or Belgian) bleached (Chicory)	
trimmed, 1 lb	68
1 head (6″)	8
1 small leave	½
chopped, 1 cup	14
Escarole	
whole, 1 lb	80
large outer leaf	5
small inner leaf	½
chopped, 1 cup	10
Fennel, raw	
whole, 1 lb	120
trimmed, 2 oz	15
Figs, raw	
whole, 1 lb	360
1 medium (2¼″)	40
dried	
8 oz	620
1 medium (2″)	58
Garlic, raw	
whole, 2 oz	68
peeled	
2 oz	80
1 clove	3

Ginger root
whole, 1 lb	205
peeled, 1 oz	14

Green (Snap) Beans, 1 cup 31

Gooseberries
1 lb	177
1 cup	59

Grapefruit
pink
whole, 1 lb	89
sections, 1 cup	80

white
whole, 1 lb	86
sections, 1 cup	80

Grapes
American slipskin: Concord, Delaware, Niagara
whole, 1 lb	197

seeded
1 cup	70
1 grape	2

European close skin: Malaga, Muscat, Thompson
whole, 1 lb	270
seeded, 1 cup	100

seedless
1 cup	107
1 grape	3½

Ground-cherries, raw
whole, 1 lb	220

without husks
1 lb	240
1 cup	74

Guava
whole, 1 lb	275
trimmed, 8 oz	140
1 average	58

Honeydew Melon
whole, 1 lb	94
cubed, 1 cup	56

8

Jack Fruit
whole, 1 lb	125
peeled and seeded, 8 oz	110

Jujubes (Chinese dates)
fresh
whole, 1 lb	444
seeded, 8 oz	238

dried
whole, 1 lb	1,160
seeded, 8 oz	650

Kale
raw
whole, 1 lb	129
without stems, 1 lb	155
leaves only, 4 oz	80

boiled, drained
1 cup	31
leaves only, 1 cup	44

Kohlrabi
raw
whole, 1 lb	96

pared
8 oz	65
diced, 1 cup	40
boiled, drained, 1 cup	40

Kumquats
whole, 1 lb	274

trimmed
8 oz	150

1 medium	12
Leeks, raw	
whole, 1 lb	123
bulb and lower leaf	
8 oz	116
1 medium	17
Lettuce	
Boston	
whole	
1 lb	47
1 head (5″)	23
1 large, 2 medium or 3 small leaves	2
chopped, 1 cup	8
Iceberg	
whole	
1 lb	56
1 head (6″)	70
1 medium leaf	3
chopped, 1 cup	7
Loose Leaf	
whole	
1 lb	52
3 large leaves	15
chopped, 1 cup	10
Romaine or cos	
whole	
1 lb	52
1 leaf	2
chopped, 1 cup	10

Limes
whole, 1 lb 106
pulp only, 1 lime 19
Loganberries
whole, 1 lb 267
trimmed
8 oz 140
1 cup 90
Loqats
whole, 1 lb 168
seeded
8 oz 110
1 medium 6
Mangoes, whole
1 lb 200
1 medium 150
1 cup 110
Mushrooms, raw
whole, 1 lb 123
chopped, 1 cup 20
Mustard Greens
raw
whole
1 lb 57
trimmed, 8 oz 70
boiled, drained, leaves only
8 oz 52
1 cup 32
Mustard Spinach (Tendergreens)
raw, whole, 1 lb 100

boiled, drained	
8 oz	37
1 cup	30
Nectarines, whole	
1 lb	267
1 medium	88
New Zealand Spinach	
raw, whole, 1 lb	86
boiled, drained	
8 oz	30
1 cup	23
Okra	
raw	
whole, 1 lb	140
trimmed, 8 oz	80
boiled, drained, sliced, 1 cup	45
Onions, mature	
raw	
whole, 1 lb	157
trimmed	
8 oz	85
1 medium	40
chopped, 1 cup	65
chopped, 1 Tbsp	4
grated, 1 cup	90
boiled, drained, 1 cup	60
Onions, young green	
whole, 1 lb	157
bulb and top	
trimmed, 1 lb	164

chopped, 1 cup	36
chopped, 1 Tbsp	2
top only, chopped	
1 cup	27
1 Tbsp	2

Onions, Welsh
raw

whole, 1 lb	100
trimmed, 8 oz	78

Oranges
whole

1 lb	162
1 medium	64
diced, 1 cup	103

Papaw
whole

1 lb	290
1 medium	83
peeled and seeded	
8 oz	185
1 cup	210

Papayas
whole

1 lb	120
1 medium	120
peeled and seeded	
8 oz	90
cubed, 1 cup	55

Parsley

whole, 1 lb	200
chopped	
1 cup	26
1 Tbsp	2
1 sprig	4

Parsnips

raw, whole, 1 lb	293
boiled, drained	
diced, 1 cup	100
mashed, 1 cup	140

Passion Fruit

whole	
1 lb	210
1 medium	15
shelled, 8 oz	200

Peaches

whole, 1 lb	150
peeled, 1 medium	38
pared, diced, 1 cup	70

Pears, 1 pear

Bartlett	200
Bosc	85
D'Anjou	120

Peas, green immature

raw	
whole, 1 lb	150
shelled	
1 lb	380
1 cup	120

boiled, drained

8 oz	160
1 cup	115

Peas, mature, dried

raw

whole

1 lb	1,540
1 cup	680
split, uncoated, 1 cup	700
cooked, split, uncoated, 1 cup	230

Pea Pods (Snow Peas)

whole, 1 lb	228

Pepper, Hot chili, green, raw

whole, 1 lb	120
seeded, 8 oz	85

Pepper, Hot chili, red

raw

whole, 1 lb	400
seeded, 8 oz	145
pods, dried, 1 Tbsp	25

Peppers, Sweet, green, raw

whole

1 lb	80
1 pepper, fancy grade large	35
1 pepper, No 1 grade	15
chopped, 1 cup	33

Peppers, Sweet, red, raw

whole, 1 lb	110
seeded and cored, 8 oz	70
chopped, 1 cup	47

Persimmon
Japanese or Kaki
  whole, 1 lb   286
  seedless, 1 lb   295
  trimmed, 1 medium   130
native
  whole
    1 lb   475
    1 medium   32
  trimmed and seeded, 8 oz   65

Pigeon peas
raw, whole, 1 lb   210
dried, 8 oz   760

Pineapple
whole, 1 lb   125
cubed, 1 cup   80

Pitanga (Surinam Cherries)
whole
  1 lb   187
  4 medium   10
pitted, 1 cup   87

Plantains, raw
whole, 1 lb   390
peeled, 8 oz   270
1 banana (10″)   285

Plums
Damson
  whole
    1 lb   272

1 medium	7
pitted, 8 oz	150
Japanese	
whole	
1 lb	205
1 medium	32
pitted, 8 oz	110
Prune type	
whole	
1 lb	320
1 medium	21
pitted, 8 oz	170
Poke Shoot (Pokeberry)	
raw, 1 lb	104
boiled, drained, 1 cup	33
Pomegranate	
whole	
1 lb	194
1 medium	100
Potatoes	
raw	
whole, 1 lb	280
peeled, 1 cup	114
baked in skin	
4 oz	81
1 long	145
boiled in skin	
4 oz	79
1 long	173
1 round	104

8

boiled, peeled

4 oz	74
1 cup	100

fried, 4 oz 275

hash brown, 4 oz 260

mashed, with milk and butter

4 oz	107
1 cup	137

scalloped, with cheese, 4 oz 118

Prickly Pears, raw

whole, 1 lb	84
peeled and seeded, 8 oz	96

Prunes, dehydrated, uncooked

8 oz	780
1 cup	344

Pumpkin, raw

whole, 1 lb	83
pulp only, 8 oz	60

Purslane leaves

raw, whole, 1 lb	95
boiled, drained, 1 cup	27

Quinces

whole, 1 lb	158
peeled and seeded, 8 oz	130

Radishes, raw

whole

1 lb	49
10 medium	8

sliced, 1 cup 20

Radishes, Oriental

whole, 1 lb	57
without tops, 1 lb	67
pared, 8 oz	45

Raisins, seedless

8 oz	655
1 cup loose	420
1 cup firmly packed	477

Raspberries

black

1 lb	330
1 cup	98

red

1 lb	260
1 cup	70

Rhubarb

raw

whole, 1 lb	33
trimmed, 1 lb	60
diced, 1 cup	20
cooked, sweetened, 1 cup	381

Rose Apples

whole, 1 lb	170
trimmed and seeded, 8 oz	138

Rutabagas

raw

whole, 1 lb	177
trimmed, 8 oz	105
diced, 1 cup	60

boiled, drained	
cubes, 1 cup	60
mashed, 1 cup	84
Sapodillas	
whole, 1 lb	323
peeled and seeded, 8 oz	202
Shallots, raw	
whole, 1 oz	18
peeled	
1 oz	20
1 Tbsp	7
Soursop, raw	
whole, 1 lb	200
peeled and seeded, 8 oz	149
Soybean curd (Tofu)	
4 oz	82
Spinach	
raw	
whole, 1 lb	85
trimmed	
leaves, 1 cup	9
chopped, 1 cup	14
boiled, drained, leaves, 1 cup	41
Squash, summer	
raw	
whole, 1 lb	85
trimmed, 8 oz	25
diced, 1 cup	35
boiled, drained, 1 cup	30

Squash, winter

raw, whole, 1 lb	150
baked, 8 oz	120

Strawberries, whole

1 lb	161
trimmed, 1 lb	168
1 cup	55

Sugar Apples (Sweetsop)

whole, 1 lb	192
peeled and seeded	
8 oz	220
1 cup	235

Swamp Cabbage

raw	
whole, 1 lb	107
trimmed, 1 lb	132
boiled, drained, 8 oz	48

Sweet Potatoes

raw, whole, 1 lb	420
baked in skin, 4 oz	125

Tamarinds

whole, 1 lb	520
shelled and seeded, 8 oz	540

Tomatoes, green

whole, 1 lb	99

Tomatoes, ripe

raw	
whole	
1 lb	100
1 medium	25

8

sliced, 1 cup	40
boiled, 1 cup	63
Towel Gourd	
whole, 1 lb	70
pared, 8 oz	40
Turnip Greens	
raw	
whole, 1 lb	107
trimmed, 1 lb	127
boiled	
8 oz	46
1 cup	30
Turnips	
raw	
whole, 1 lb	117
cubed, 1 cup	39
boiled, drained	
8 oz	52
1 cup	36
mashed	53
Vinespinach (Basella), raw, 8 oz	44
Water Chestnuts, Chinese	
raw, whole, 1 lb	276
Watercress	
whole	
1 lb	80
1 cup	7
chopped, 1 cup	24
Watermelon	
whole, 1 lb	54

8

1 wedge (4″ x 8″)	110
diced, 1 cup	42
Wax (Yellow) Beans	
1 cup	29
Yam Beans, raw	
whole, 1 lb	225
pared, 8 oz	130
Yams, raw	
whole, 1 lb	395
pared, 4 oz	115
Zucchini (see Summer Squash)	

FRUIT,
COMMERCIALLY PACKAGED,
CANNED OR FROZEN,
½ cup unless noted

Apples and Apricots	
Mott's	104
Apples and Cherries	
Mott's	110
Apples and Pineapples	
Mott's	127

Apples and Raspberries
Mott's	105

Applesauce
Del Monte	85
Mott's	45
S & W	48
Stokely-Van Camp	90
Tillie Lewis	60
Town House	85

Apricots
Del Monte	100
Libby's	100
Stokely-Van Camp	110
Tillie Lewis	60
Town House	80

Blackberries
S & W	36

Blueberries
Seabrook Farms	45

Boysenberries
S & W	32

Cherries
Del Monte Light	95
Dark	90
Dark pitted	95
Libby's	100
S & W	50
Stokely-Van Camp	50

Cherries, maraschino
Vita 1 cherry	20

Cranberry and Orange
  Ocean Spray   100
Cranberry Sauce
  Ocean Spray   90
Currants
  Del Monte   190
Dates
  Bordo   330
  Dromedary   397
  Dromedary pitted   376
Figs
  Del Monte   100
  S & W, 6 figs   49
Fruit Cocktail
  Del Monte   85
  Dole   72
  Libby's   75
  S & W   35
  Stokely-Van Camp   95
  Tillie Lewis   50
  Town House   85
Fruit Salad
  Del Monte   85
  Del Monte Tropical   100
  Kraft   48
  Libby's   90
  S & W   35
  Stokely-Van Camp   95
Fruits and Peels
  Liberty   388

Grapefruit sections
Del Monte	45
Kraft	43
S & W	36
Tillie Lewis	45

Mixed Fruit
Birds Eye	105

Melon Balls
Birds Eye, 1 pkg	144

Oranges
Del Monte	75
Kraft	52
S & W	27

Peaches
Birds Eye	72
Del Monte	85
Highway	70
S & W	25
Scotch Buy	70
Seabrook Farms	105
Stokely-Van Camp	90
Town House, heavy syrup	95
Town House, extra heavy syrup	130

Peaches and Strawberries
Birds Eye	80

Pears
Del Monte	80
Libby's	85
Libby's Juice Pack	75
Highway	80

Scotch Buy   70
S & W   28
Stokely-Van Camp   105
Tillie Lewis   50

Pineapple
Del Monte in juice   70
Del Monte in syrup   95
Dole in juice   65
Dole in syrup   85
S & W   50
Town House in juice   75
Town House in syrup   95

Plums
Del Monte   95
Libby's   105
S & W   50
Stokely-Van Camp   120
Tillie Lewis   70

Prunes
Del Monte   115
Heart's Delight   210
Sunsweet   196

Raspberries
Birds Eye   120
Seabrook Farms   120

Rhubarb
Birds Eye   138

Strawberries
Birds Eye   90
Birds Eye slices   145

Seabrook Farms	42
Seabrook Farms slices	140
S & W	20

VEGETABLES, COMMERCIALLY PACKAGED, CANNED OR FROZEN,
1 cup unless noted

Artichoke Hearts	
Birds Eye	53
Asparagus, cuts	
Green Giant	40
Kounty Kist	40
Lindy	39
Stokely-Van Camp	44
Asparagus, Spears	
Del Monte	35
Green Giant	40
Le Sueur	38
S & W	18
Town House	35
Asparagus, frozen	
Birds Eye	61
with Hollandaise Sauce, 1 pkg	290

Green Giant	90
Seabrook Farms	46
Bamboo Shoots	
Chun King	30
La Choy	23
Bean Sprouts	
Chun King	40
La Choy	24
Beets, cut	
Del Monte	70
Libby's	70
Stokely-Van Camp	90
Beets, diced	
Comstock	82
Libby's	70
Stokely-Van Camp	70
Beets, Harvard	
Greenwood	104
Libby's	160
Lord Mott	80
Stokely-Van Camp	160
Beets, pickled	
Del Monte	150
Greenwood	150
Libby's	150
Lord Mott	150
Stokely-Van Camp	190
Town House	145
Beets, sliced	
Del Monte	70

8

Libby's	70
Lord Mott	50
S & W	56
Stokely-Van Camp	80
Beets, whole	
Del Monte	70
Libby's	70
Stokely-Van Camp	85
Beets, frozen	
Birds Eye	105
Broccoli, frozen	
Birds Eye	25
with cheese	110
in hollandaise	200
Green Giant	30
in butter	90
in cheese sauce	130
with cauliflower and carrots	140
Kounty Kist	30
Seabrook Farms	46
Stouffer's Au gratin	340
Brussels Sprouts	
Birds Eye	30
Green Giant	50
in butter sauce	110
in cheese sauce	170
Kounty Kist	50
Seabrook Farms	76
Cabbage	
Greenwood	150

Lord Mott	120
Carrots, diced	
Comstock	48
Del Monte	61
Libby's	40
S & W	44
Stokely-Van Camp	60
Carrots, sliced	
Birds Eye, in buttersauce	340
in sugar	194
Comstock	35
Del Monte	58
Green Giant, in butter sauce	100
Libby's	42
Lord Mott	50
Stokely-Van Camp	50
Cauliflower	
Birds Eye	61
with cheese sauce	130
Green Giant	30
with cheese sauce	130
Kounty Kist	26
Seabrook Farms	26
Collard Greens	
Birds Eye	30
Seabrook Farms	44
Corn, Yellow, canned	
cream style	
Birds Eye	170
Del Monte	210

Green Giant	210
S & W	168
Stokely-Van Camp	210
liquid pack	
Del Monte	170
Green Giant	160
Kounty Kist	180
Le Sueur	170
Libby's	160
S & W	104
Stokely-Van Camp	180
vacuum pack	
Del Monte	200
Green Giant	160
Kounty Kist	160
Stokely-Van Camp	240
with peppers	
Del Monte	190
Green Giant	150
Corn, Yellow, frozen	
Birds Eye in butter sauce	200
Green Giant in butter sauce	190
with peppers	180
Stouffer's, 1 pkg	465
Corn, White, frozen and canned	
Birds Eye creamed	170
with peas	140
Del Monte creamed	190
kernels	150
Green Giant	130

Kounty Kist	140
Eggplant Parmesan	
Mrs. Paul's	364
Eggplant slices	
Mrs. Paul's	613
Eggplant sticks	
Mrs. Paul's	254
Kale	
Seabrook Farms	60
Mixed Vegetables, canned	
Del Monte	79
La Choy	35
Libby's	78
Stokely-Van Camp	81
Town House	88
Mixed Vegetables, frozen	
Birds Eye	145
Chun King	23
Green Giant	90
Kounty Kist	89
California	30
La Choy	23
Mixed Vegetables, frozen, Chinese style	
Birds Eye Cantonese	123
Birds Eye International	48
Green Giant	130
La Choy	72
Mixed Vegetables, frozen, European styles	
Birds Eye	
Danish	74

Italian	98
Parisian	74

Mixed Vegetables, frozen, Hawaiian style

Birds Eye	98
Green Giant	197

Mixed Vegetables, frozen, Japanese style

Birds Eye	98
Birds Eye with seasonings	74
Green Giant	130
La Choy, 1 pkg	71

Mixed Vegetables, frozen, American styles

Birds Eye

New England	150
New Orleans Creole	150
Jubilee	250
Pennsylvania Dutch	98
San Francisco	111
Wisconsin	111
Green Giant	130

Mushrooms

Birds Eye	50
Brandywine	30
B & B	60
Dole	5
Green Giant	15

Mustard greens

Birds Eye	44
Seabrook Farms	42

Okra

Birds Eye	61

Green Giant	211
Seabrook Farms	52
Onions	
Birds Eye	64
in cream sauce	239
whole	98
Green Giant	140
Lord Mott	60
in cream sauce	130
Ore-Ida	80
Seabrook Farms	232
Onion Rings, 1 oz	
Birds Eye	170
Mrs. Paul's	60
O & C	178
Ore-Ida	80
Peas, canned	
early	
Del Monte	110
Kounty Kist	139
Le Sueur	110
Lindy	138
Lord Mott	110
Minnesota Valley	109
Stokely-Van Camp	128
sweet	
Del Monte	101
Green Giant	110
with onion	105
Kounty Kist	131

Libby's	121
Lindy	130
S & W	70
Stokely-Van Camp	130
with carrots	
Del Monte	100
Libby's	101
Lord Mott	165
S & W	65
Stokely-Van Camp	120
Peas, frozen	
early	
Birds Eye	169
Green Giant	102
Kounty Kist	119
Le Sueur	149
Seabrook Farms	148
sweet	
Birds Eye	155
Green Giant	150
Seabrook Farms	104
with carrots	
Birds Eye	122
Kounty Kist	90
Seabrook Farms	82
with cream sauce	
Birds Eye	369
Green Giant	300
with cream sauce and cauliflower	
Birds Eye	247

in onion sauce
   Seabrook Farms — 192
with onions
   Birds Eye — 149
with onions and carrots
   Le Sueur — 180
with potatos
   Birds Eye — 431
with mushrooms
   Birds Eye — 155

Peppers, green
   Stouffers, 1 pkg — 225
   Weight Watchers, one 13-oz pkg — 320

Potatoes, canned
   Del Monte — 90
   Hormel au gratin, 7½-oz can — 270
     with ham, 7½-oz can — 255
   Stokely-Van Camp — 103

Potatoes, frozen, 3 oz unless noted
   Au gratin
     Green Giant, 1 cup — 390
     Stouffer's — 270
   French fried
     Birds Eye
       Crinkle Cuts — 124
       Cottage Fries — 120
       Gold Crinkle Cuts — 140
       French — 111
       Shoestrings — 138
       Steak Fries — 109

Ore-Ida

Cottage Fries	140
Golden Crinkles	130
Sizzling Fries	157
Sizzling Crinkles	171
Sizzling Shoestrings	218
Shoestrings	170

Hash browns

Birds Eye	54
O'Brien	45
Ore-Ida	70
in butter sauce	120
in butter sauce and onions	130

with parsley

Seabrook Farms	208

Scalloped

Stouffer's	252

Shredded hash browns

Birds Eye	60
Ore-Ida	60

Slices

Green Giant	210

with sour cream

Green Giant	270

Stuffed

Green Giant

with cheese, 5 oz	240
with sour cream, 5 oz	229

with peas

Green Giant	242

Taters and Puffs
Birds Eye Tasti Fries	140
Tasti Puffs	190
Ore-Ida Tater Tots	160
Tater Tots with Bacon	151
Tater Tots with Onion	165

With Vermicelli
Green Giant	399

Whole
Birds Eye	179
Ore-Ida	70
Seabrook Farms	153

Potatoes, mix, ½ cup
French's	120
Big Tate	129
Hungry Jack	160

Julienne
Betty Crocker	132

Au gratin
Betty Crocker	150
French's	190

Creamed
Betty Crocker	163

Hash browns
Betty Crocker	147
French's	160

Pancakes
French's 3 cakes	130

Potato Buds
Betty Crocker	132

Scalloped
  Betty Crocker 150
  French's 189
With sour cream
  Betty Crocker 144

Pumpkin
  Del Monte 79
  Libby's 80
  Stokely-Van Camp 88

Sauerkraut
  Del Monte 50
  Libby's 42
  Stokely-Van Camp 50
    Bavarian 69

Soup Greens
  Durkee 213

Spinach, canned
  Del Monte 45
  Libby's 44
  Lord Mott 44

Spinach, frozen
  chopped
    Birds Eye 47
    Seabrook Farms 50
  creamed
    Birds Eye 157
    Green Giant 190
    Lord Mott 130

Seabrook Farms	200
leaf	
Birds Eye	47
Seabrook Farms	48
souffle	
Green Giant	300
Stouffer's, 1 pkg	400
with butter sauce	
Green Giant	89
Squash	
Birds Eye	100
Green Giant	118
Seabrook Farms	92
Stew, vegetable	
Dinty Moore, 7½-oz can	160
Ore-Ida	140
Succotash	
Birds Eye	202
Libby's creamed	190
kernel	151
Seabrook Farms	174
Stokely-Van Camp	170
Sweet Potatoes	
Birds Eye	408
Green Giant	341
Lord Mott	235
Mrs. Paul's	320
Tomatoes	
stewed	70
whole	50

Tomato paste
   Contadina   200
   Del Monte   200
   Hunt's   185
   Town House   225

Tomato puree
   Contadina   120

Turnip Greens
   Birds Eye   47
   Seabrook Farms   44
   Stokely-Van Camp   46

Zucchini
   Birds Eye   39
   Del Monte   60
   Mrs. Paul's   480

CHAPTER 9

Condiments, Dips, Dressings, Oils and Sauces

CONDIMENTS,
1 Tbsp, unless noted

celery flakes, 1 tsp
   Wyler's   7
curry powder
   Crosse & Blackwell   26
garlic flavoring, 1 tsp
   Burton's   42
garlic powder, 1 tsp
   Wyler's   8
garlic spread
   Lawry's   88
horseradish
   Borden   16
   Heinz   26
   Kraft   4
   Tastee   5
hot sauce, 1 tsp
   Frank's   10
   Gebhardt   4
   Tabasco   4
meat sauces
   A-1   12
   Crosse & Blackwell   21
   Durkee   60
   Escoffier   19
   Gravymaster, 1 tsp   8
   Heinz 57   14
   Heinz Savory   21
   H.P.   21
   Maggi   17

Steak Supreme	20
mustard	
Brown	
French's	15
Gulden's	13
Heinz	11
Mr. Mustard	11
Dijon	
Grey Poupon	15
German	
Kraft	15
Horseradish	
French's	15
Hot	
Gulden's Diablo	13
Heinz	11
Onion	
French's	25
Yellow	
French's	16
Gulden's	11
Heinz	10
Kraft	12
onion flakes, 1 tsp	
Wyler's	7
onion flavoring, 1 tsp	
Burton's	42
onion powder, 1 tsp	
Wyler's	1

onions, minced, 1 tsp
  Borden's   7
  Wyler's   7
parsley flakes, 1 tsp
  Wyler's   1
pepper
  Seasoned
    Lawry's, 1 tsp   16
  sweet
    Wyler's, 1 tsp   2
salt, flavored, 1 tsp
  celery   6
  garlic   6
  onion   6
sandwich spread
  Hellman's   60
  Kraft   56
vinegar
  Cider or white   1
  Wine
    Holland House
      Marsala   35
      Red   25
      Sherry   40
      White   25
    Regina
      Sauterne   1
      Sherry   10

Flavorings, Extracts, 1 tsp

Almond
  Durkee   13
  Ehlers   5
Anise
  Durkee   16
  Ehlers   12
Banana
  Durkee   15
  Ehlers   7
Black Walnut
  Durkee   45
Brandy
  Durkee   15
  Ehlers   18
Cherry
  Ehlers   8
Chocolate
  Durkee   8
Coconut
  Durkee   7
  Ehlers   13
Lemon
  Durkee   17
  Ehlers   14
Maple
  Durkee   6
  Ehlers   9

Mocha
   Durkee   14
Orange
   Durkee   16
   Ehlers   14
Peppermint
   Durkee   15
   Ehlers   12
Pineapple
   Ehlers   13
Raspberry
   Ehlers   10
Rum
   Durkee   14
   Ehlers   12
Strawberry
   Durkee   12
   Ehlers   11
Vanilla
   Durkee   5

Relishes, Pickles, Olives:
1 piece unless noted

Capers, 1 Tbsp
   Crosse & Blackwell   6

Carrots, dill
  Cresca Cocktail Sticks   1
Cauliflower, sweet
  Heinz   9
  Smucker's   23
ChowChow, 1 Tbsp
  Crosse & Blackwell   20
Chutney
  Major Grey's   53
Eggplant
  Cresca   1
Olives
  Green, Manzanilla
    Durkee   4
    Grandee   4
  Green, Spanish
    Vita   11
  Green, queen
    Durkee   14
    Grandee   14
  Ripe
    Durkee   7
    Grandee   7
    Lindsay   6
    Vita   7
Onions
  Cresca   1
  Crosse & Blackwell   1
  Heinz   2
  Heinz Spiced   1

Peppers, 1 oz unless noted
  Chili
    Del Monte 5
    Ortega
      Jalapeños 8
      Green 5
  Hot, 1 pepper
    Cresca 6
    Smucker's 10
  Mild, sweet
    Del Monte 5
  Pickled
    Old El Paso 9
  Red, bell
    Ortega 9
Pickle Relish, 1 Tbsp
  Barbecue
    Crosse & Blackwell 22
    Heinz 31
  Corn
    Crosse & Blackwell 15
  Hamburger
    Crosse & Blackwell 20
    Heinz 17
  Hot dog
    Crosse & Blackwell 22
    Heinz 2
  Hot pepper
    Crosse & Blackwell 22

India
   Crosse & Blackwell   26
piccalilli
   Crosse & Blackwell   25
   Heinz   19

Pickles
  Sour
    Bond's   2
    Crosse & Blackwell   2
    Heinz
      Genuine Dill   10
      Kosher Dills   2
    L & S   2
  Sweet
    Bond's   19
    Crosse & Blackwell   28
      slices, 1 Tbsp   15
    Heinz
      Midget   5
      Sweet Gherkins   25
      Sweet Pickles   45
      Sticks   13
      Candied dill strips   35

Pimientos, 1 oz
  Dromedary   8
  Ortega   7
  Stokely-Van Camp   8
Watermelon Rind, 1 Tbsp   38

Seasonings, 1 tsp unless noted

Accent	9
Bacon	
Ann Page	8
Baco's	13
Durkee	3
French's	2
Lawry's	13
McCormick	
Bits	10
Chips	12
Schilling	
Bits	19
Chips	13
Barbecue	
French's	6
Chili Powder	
Lawry's	9
Mexene	8
Cinnamon Sugar	
French's	16
Chutney	
Major Grey's	16
Spice Island	12
Herb	
Lawry's	9
Horseradish	
Reese	18

9

Hot Sauce
Frank's — 1
Lemon Pepper
Lawry's — 7
French's — 6
Meat Tenderizer
French's — 2
Pepper
French's — 8
Lawry's — 8
Salad
Durkee — 4
  with cheese — 10
French's — 6
Salt
French's
  Butter — 8
  Celery — 2
  Garlic — 4
  Hickory Smoked — 2
  Onion — 6
  Parsley Garlic — 6
  Seasoned — 2
Lawry's
  Garlic — 5
  Onion — 4
  Seasoned — 1
Seafood
French's — 2

Stock Base
  French's   8

Seasoning Mixes, 1 pkg, various sizes

A la King
  Durkee   297
Beef
  Lawry's
    Beef Olé   126
    Marinade   69
Beef Stew
  Durkee   99
  French's   150
  Lawry's   131
  McCormick   90
  Schilling   89
Beef Stroganoff
  French's   192
  Lawry's   119
  McCormick   113
Beef, Ground
  Ann Page   100
  Durkee   91
  French's   100
Chili
  Ann Page   120
  French's   150

Pizza	99
French's	128
Lawry's	139
McCormick	167
Schilling	172
Rice, Fried	
Durkee	62
Rice, Spanish	
Durkee	129
Lawry's	125
Swiss Steak	
McCormick	44
Schilling	42
Taco	
Durkee	67
French's	150
McCormick	65
Schilling	65
Tuna Casserole	
McCormick	104

DIPS, 1 oz

Ready to Serve

Bacon and Horseradish
  Borden   79
  Kraft
    Ready   71
    Teez   57
  Lucerne   63
Bacon and Smoke
  Sealtest   47
Barbecue
  Borden's   48
Bean
  Chili
    Lucerne   50
  Jalapeño
    Frito-Lay   36
    Gebhardt   30
    Granny Goose   37
    Lucerne   35
Blue Cheese
  Granny Goose   110
  Kraft
    Ready   69
    Teez   51

Lucerne 67

Sealtest 49

Casino

Sealtest 45

Chili, Green

Borden 55

Chipped Beef

Sealtest 44

Clam

Kraft

Ready 66

Teez 44

Lucerne 34

Clam and Lobster

Borden 60

Dill

Kraft 67

Garlic

Granny Goose 100

Kraft 47

Lucerne 58

Green Goddess

Kraft 45

Guacamole

Lucerne 69

Hickory Smoke

Lucerne 60

Onion

Borden 48

Lawry's 50

Kraft	
Ready	68
Teez	43
Lucerne	58
Sealtest	46
Tartar	
Borden	48

Unprepared Mixes

Bacon and Onion	
Frito-Lay	100
Barbecue	
Salada	120
Blue Cheese	
Frito-Lay	117
Lawry's	94
Caesar	
Frito-Lay	118
Lawry's	94
Cheddar Cheese	
Salada	43
Chili	
Frito-Lay	120
Dill	
Frito-Lay	90
Dill and Chives	
Salada	130

Garlic and Onion
  McCormick   126
  Salada   100
Horseradish
  Lawry's   86
  Frito-Lay   105
Onion
  Frito-Lay   87
    Green   100
  Lawry's
    Green   100
    Toasted   82
  McCormick   131
  Salada   100
Taco
  Frito-Lay   105

SALAD DRESSINGS,
1 Tbsp unless noted

Avocado
  Kraft   70
Bacon
  Lawry's   78
Blue Cheese
  Ann Page Low Calorie   18

Kraft
    Chunky   70
    Low Calorie   14
    Low Calorie Chunky   30
Lawry's
    bottled   57
    mix, 1 pkg   74
Nu Made   75
Roka   60
Seven Seas   70
Wish-Bone   80
Weight Watchers   10
Caesar
Kraft   70
Lawry's
    bottled   70
    mix, 1 pkg   72
Nu Made   75
Pfeiffer   70
    Low Calorie   10
Seven Seas   70
Wish-Bone   80
Chef Style
Ann Page   20
Kraft   18
Coach House
Seven Seas   78
Coleslaw
Kraft   70
    Low Calorie   30

Cucumber

Kraft 80

  Low Calorie 30

French

Ann Page 25

Casino 70

Kraft 60

  Casino Garlic 70

  Herb and Garlic 90

  Low Calorie 25

  Miracle 70

Lawry's

  bottled 50

  mix, 1 pkg 72

Nu Made

  Low Calorie 20

  Savory 65

  Zesty 70

Pfeiffer 55

  Low Calorie 18

Seven Seas 60

  Low Calorie 30

Tillie Lewis 12

Wish-Bone

  Deluxe 50

  French Garlic 70

  Low Calorie 25

  Sweet and Spicy 70

Weight Watchers 4

Garlic
Kraft	50
Wish-Bone	80

Green Goddess
Kraft	80
Lawry's	
bottled	60
mix, 1 pkg	69
Nu Made	80
Seven Seas	80
Wish-Bone	60

Green Onion
Kraft	70

Hawaiian
Lawry's	75

Herb and Garlic
Kraft	83

Herb and Spices
Seven Seas	60

Italian
Ann Page	14
Good Seasons	8
Kraft	80
Golden	70
Low Calorie	6
Lawry's	
bottled	80
mix, 1 pkg	44
cheeses mix, 1 pkg	69

Nu Made	90
Low Calorie	16
Pfeiffer	60
Low Calorie	10
Seven Seas	70
Family	60
Low Calorie	35
Viva	70
Tillie Lewis	6
Weight Watchers	2
Wish-Bone	80
Low Calorie	20
Lemon garlic	
Lawry's, 1 pkg	65
Mayonnaise, all brands	100
Mayonnaise, flavored	
Durkee	69
Mayonnaise, imitation	
Mrs. Filbert's	40
Piedmont	50
Weight Watchers	40
May Lo Naise	
Tillie Lewis	25
Oil and Vinegar	
Kraft	70
Lawry's	55
Nu Made	60
Seven Seasons	70
Onion	
Lawry's	84

Wish-Bone	80
Parmesan	
Good Seasons	84
Roquefort	
Kraft	58
Red Wine	
Pfeiffer	40
Low Calorie	10
Russian	
Kraft	30
Nu Made	55
Pfeiffer	65
Low Calorie	15
Seven Seas	80
Tillie Lewis	12
Weight Watchers	
bottled	50
mix	4
Wish-Bone	60
Low Calorie	25
Salad dressing	
Ann Page	70
Heinz	63
Kraft	65
Mrs. Filbert's	65
Nu Made	80
Piedmont	70
Sultana	50
Salad Secret	
Kraft	60

Sea Island
Kraft   93
Sour Treat
Friendship   90
Sherry
Lawry's   55
Spin Blend
Hellmann's   55
Tahitian Isle
Wish-Bone   55
Thousand Island
Ann Page   25
Kraft   60
   Low Calorie   30
Lawry's
   bottled   65
   mix, 1 pkg   78
Nu Made   30
Pfeiffer   65
   Low Calorie   15
Seven Seas   50
Tillie Lewis   18
Weight Watchers
   bottled   50
   mix   12
Wish-Bone   70
   Low Calorie   25
Tomato-Blue Cheese
Kraft   90

Tomato-Spice
  Seven Seas — 45
Whipped
  Tillie Lewis — 25
Yogonaise
  Henri's — 60
Yogowhip
  Henri's — 60
Yogurt, all flavors
  Henri's — 35

OILS, 1 Tbsp

Corn
  Mazola — 122
  Nu Made — 124
Olive
  Filippo Berio — 125
Peanut
  Planters — 128
Popcorn
  Planters — 130
Safflower
  Nu Made — 119
Soybean
  Mrs. Tucker's — 128

Sunflower
 Sunlight   120
Vegetable
 Crisco   120
 Puritan   118
 Swift   115
 Wesson   120
Vegetable and cottonseed
 Swift   120

Shortening, 1 Tbsp unless noted

Lard   115
 1 cup   1,850
Vegetable
 Crisco   109
 Fluffo   109
 Mrs. Tucker's   120
 Pam   7
 Snowdrift   111
 Spry   97

SAUCES,
½ cup unless noted

A la King
Durkee	66

Barbecue, 1 Tbsp
Chris' and Pitt's	15
Durkee with vinegar	64
French's	14
Hot	27
Smoky	14
Open Pit	26
Hot 'n Spicy	27
Hickory Smoked	27
with onions	28

Bearnaise
Butternut Farm	176

Bordelaise
Butternut Farm	48

Cheese
Durkee	168
French's	160
McCormick	156
Schilling	156

Chili
Gebhardt	156
Heinz	17

Hunt's	18
McCormick	92
Clam	
Buitoni	
red	102
white	114
La Rosa	
red	78
white	68
Cocktail Sauce	
Crosse & Blackwell	26
Tastee	25
Enchilada	
Gebhardt	68
Lawry's, 1 pkg	144
McCormick, 1 pkg	116
Old El Paso	
Hot	36
Mild	40
Hollandaise	
Durkee	118
French's	119
McCormick	171
Schilling	170
Horseradish, 1 oz	
Kraft	100
Italian	
Contadina	85
Lawry's, 1 pkg	86
Ragu	36

Lemon-Butter, 1 oz
Weight Watchers 16
Mint Sauce, 1 tsp
Crosse & Blackwell 16
Mushroom, 1 oz
Dawn Fresh 9
Pizza
Buitoni 92
Ragu 96
Seafood cocktail sauce, 1 tsp
Del Monte 18
Pfeiffer 25
Sour Cream
Durkee 160
French's 280
McCormick 146
Schilling 146
Soy Sauce, 1 tsp
La Choy 7
Spaghetti
Ann Page 70
Marinara 70
Meat 80
Mix, 1 envelope 120
with Mushrooms 70
Buitoni 92
Clam, red 108
Clam, white 144
Marinara 88
Meat 120

with Mushrooms	88
Durkee	45
with Mushrooms	40
French's	80
with Mushrooms	80
Franco-American	95
with Mushrooms	95
Lawry's	147
with Meatball seasoning	316
with Mushrooms	116
La Rosa	74
Prince	90
with Meat	143
with Mushrooms	103
Ragu	
Plain	96
Thick	84
Clam	88
Marinara	96
Meat	92
Thick with Meatball seasoning	104
with Mushrooms	84
Spatini	51
Town House	80
with Meat	80
with Mushrooms	89
Stroganoff	
Durkee	410
French's	165
Lawry's, 1 pkg	118

Special	40
with Bits	35
with Cheese	71
with Herbs	80
with Meat	120
with Mushrooms	40
with Onions	45
Stokely-Van Camp	35
Town House	40
Tomato Paste	
Contadina	46
Hunt's	108
Lord Mott	44
Tuna Casserole	
McCormick	128
Schilling	128
White	
Durkee	119
Wine, 1 oz	
Lawry's	
Burgundy	98
Sherry	94
White	113
Worcestershire Sauce	
Crosse & Blackwell	15
Heinz	11
French's	10
Lea & Perrins	12

Gravies, ¼ cup unless noted

Au Jus
Ann Page 1 envelope	64
Durkee	8
Durkee, Roastin' Bag, 1 pkg	64
French's	8
French's Pan Rich	30
McCormick	4
Schilling	4

Beef
Franco-American	30
Howard Johnson's	25
Wyler's	24

Brown
Ann Page 1 envelope	79
Dawn Fresh	20
Durkee	15
with Mushrooms	15
with Onions	17
Franco-American	25
French's	20
French's Pan Rich	62
McCormick	26
Herb	21
Lite	10
Pillsbury	15
Schilling	26
Herb	21

Weight Watchers	8
with Mushrooms	12
with Onions	13
Chicken	
Ann Page, 1 envelope	120
College Inn	25
Durkee	22
Creamy	39
Roastin' Bag, 1 pkg	122
Roastin' Bag Italian, 1 pkg	144
French's	25
French's Pan Rich	60
McCormick	21
Lite	10
Pillsbury	25
Schilling	21
Lite	10
Weight Watchers	10
Wyler's	24
Chicken Giblet	
Franco-American	35
Herb	
McCormick	26
Homestyle	
Durkee	18
French's	25
Pillsbury	15
Meatloaf	
Durkee, 1 pkg	130

Mushroom
  Ann Page, 1 envelope   79
  Durkee   16
  Franco-American   35
  French's   20
  McCormick   19
  Schilling   19
  Wyler's   15

Mustard
  French's   16

Onion
  Ann Page, 1 envelope   120
  Durkee   21
  Durkee Roastin' Bag, 1 pkg   124
  French's   25
  French's Pan Rich   50

Pork
  Durkee   18
  Durkee Roastin' Bag, 1 pkg   130
  French's   20

Pot Roast
  Durkee, 1 pkg   124

Sparerib
  Durkee, 1 pkg   162

Swiss Steak
  Durkee   11
  Durkee Roastin' Bag, 1 pkg   115

Turkey
  Durkee   23

9

French's	25
McCormick	21
Schilling	22
Turkey Giblet	
Howard Johnson's	28

CHAPTER 10

Desserts, Baking and Baked Goods

BAKING MISCELLANY

Baking Powder, 1 tsp	5
Yeast, ¼ oz unless noted	
Baker's	6
Brewer's	20
Dry, active	
Fleischmann's	20
Fresh, active	
Fleischmann's .6 oz pkg	15
Household	
Fleischmann's	7
Torula	20

10

Baking Chocolate, 1 oz
Chips
Baker's	130
Hershey's	115
Nestlé	130

Ground
Ghiradelli	150

Solid
Baker's
German	140
semi-sweet	130
unsweetened	140
Ghiradelli	150
Hershey	190

Butterscotch
Nestlé chips	150

Coconut
Baker's	150

Ginger
Borden's crystallized	98
Borden's preserved	88

Peanut Butter
Reese chips	150

CAKES, FROZEN,
1 whole cake

Banana
Pepperidge Farm	1,115
Sara Lee	1,439

Banana Nut
Sara Lee	1,864

Black Forest
Sara Lee	1,625

Boston Creme
Pepperidge Farm	1,070

Cheesecake
Lambrecht	1,530
Mrs. Smith's	1,230
Sara Lee	
small	860
large	1,440
Cherry	1,280
French	2,190
Strawberry	1,280
Strawberry French	2,062

Chocolate
Pepperidge Farm	1,238
Sara Lee	1,380

Chocolate Bavarian
Sara Lee	2,250

10

Chocolate Fudge
  Pepperidge Farm   1,800
Chocolate, German
  Pepperidge Farm   1,589
  Sara Lee   1,234
Coconut
  Pepperidge Farm   1,800
Crumbcake
  Sara Lee   170
  Stouffer's
    Blueberry   211
    Chocolate Chip   225
    French   200
Cupcake
  Stouffer's
    Cream   240
    Yellow   190
Devil's Food
  Pepperidge Farm   1,800
  Sara Lee   1,496
Golden
  Pepperidge Farm   900
  Sara Lee   1,440
Lemon
  Sara Lee   2,175
Lemon Coconut
  Pepperidge Farm   1,100
Mandarin Orange
  Sara Lee   1,650

Orange
   Howard Johnson's   1,700
   Sara Lee   1,440
Pound
   Sara Lee
      Banana Nut   1,170
      Chocolate   1,220
      Chocolate Swirl   1,300
      Plain   1,320
      Raisin   1,270
   Pepperidge Farm
      Apple Nut   1,300
      Butter   1,300
      Carrot   1,600
      Chocolate   1,300
Cherry
   Mrs. Smith's   2,335
Strawberry
   Mrs. Smith's   1,830
   Sara Lee   1,550
      Strawberry and Cream   1,700
Vanilla
   Pepperidge Farm   1,900
Walnut
   Sara Lee   1,690

CAKE MIXES, 1 whole cake

Angel Food
Betty Crocker	1,560
One Step	1,680
Confetti	1,800
Strawberry	1,800
Duncan Hines	1,670
Pillsbury	1,680
Swans Down	1,590

Apple Raisin
Duncan Hines	2,280
Spicy	1,620

Applesauce Raisin
Betty Crocker	1,800

Banana
Betty Crocker	3,140
Duncan Hines	2,400
Pillsbury	3,120

Banana Nut
Betty Crocker	1,800
Duncan Hines	1,800

Bundt
Pillsbury	
Fudge	3,480
Lemon	3,350
Macaroon	3,950
Marble	3,960

Pound	3,710
Triple Fudge	3,590
Butter	
Duncan Hines	3,240
Pillsbury	2,680
Butter Brickle	
Betty Crocker	3,110
Butter Fudge	
Duncan Hines	3,240
Butter Pecan	
Betty Crocker	3,120
Cheesecake	
Jello-O	2,000
Pillsbury	3,120
Royal	1,840
Cherry	
Duncan Hines	2,280
Cherry Chip	
Betty Crocker	2,280
Chocolate	
Betty Crocker	1,380
Duncan Hines	2,400
Pillsbury Dark	3,120
Swans Down	2,240
Chocolate Almond	
Betty Crocker	1,890
Chocolate Chip	
Betty Crocker	1,980
Duncan Hines	1,710
Double Chocolate Chip	1,620

Chocolate Fudge
   Betty Crocker   3,240
Chocolate, German
   Betty Crocker   3,240
   Pillsbury   3,120
Chocolate, Sour Cream
   Betty Crocker   3,240
   Duncan Hines   2,400
Chocolate, Swiss
   Duncan Hines   2,400
   Swans Down   2,240
Chocolate with frosting
   Betty Crocker   1,620
Coconut Pecan
   Betty Crocker   1,975
Date Nut
   Betty Crocker   1,890
Devil's Food
   Betty Crocker   3,240
   Duncan Hines   2,400
   Pillsbury   3,240
   Swans Down   2,230
Fudge Marble
   Duncan Hines   2,400
   Pillsbury   3,240
Gingerbread
   Betty Crocker   1,890
Lemon
   Betty Crocker   3,240
   Pudding Cake   1,380

Duncan Hines	2,400
Pillsbury	3,240

Lemon Chiffon
Betty Crocker	2,280

Marble
Betty Crocker	3,280

Orange
Betty Crocker	3,240
Duncan Hines	2,400

Pineapple
Betty Crocker	2,400
Duncan Hines	2,400

Pound
Betty Crocker	2,280

Spice
Betty Crocker	3,240
Duncan Hines	2,400

Spice Raisin
Betty Crocker	1,800

Strawberry
Betty Crocker	3,240
Duncan Hines	2,400

Streusel
Pillsbury
Cinnamon	4,080
Devil's Food	3,950
Fudge Marble	4,080
Chocolate	3,950
Lemon	4,200

10

White

Betty Crocker	2,400
Duncan Hines	2,280
Pillsbury	3,000
Swans Down	2,120

Yellow

Betty Crocker	3,240
Butter	2,880
with frosting	1,380
Duncan Hines	2,400
Pillsbury	3,120
Swans Down	2,240

CAKES FOR SNACKS, 1 cake

Big Wheels	170
Brownie	
Hostess	
small	150
large	240
Chocolate, cream-filled	
Yankee Doodles	134
Choco-Diles	250
Creamies, 1 pkg	
Tastykake	
Chocolate	255

Spice	270
Crumb Cakes	
Hostess	130
Cupcakes	
Hostess	
Chocolate	155
Orange	147
Tastykake, 1 pkg	
Buttercream	238
Chocolate	200
Chocolate Cream	239
Devil Dogs	169
Devil's Food	
Hostess	140
Drake's	135
Ding Dongs	170
Donuts	
Hostess	
Cinnamon	110
Crunch	100
Enrobed	130
Plain	105
Powdered	115
Funny Bones, 1 pkg	162
Ho-Ho's	120
Juniors, 1 pkg	
Tastykake	
Chocolate	307
Coconut	330
Coffee cake	310

10

Krimpets, 1 pkg
Tastykake
    Butterscotch   190
    Chocolate   255
    Jelly   168
    Vanilla   240

Macaroons
Hostess   210

Oatmeal Raisin, 1 pkg
Tastykake   267

Orange Treats, 1 pkg
Tastykake   230

Pound
Drake's
    Marble   185
    Plain   181
    Raisin   323

Ring Ding   366
Sno Balls   140

Tandy Takes, 1 pkg
    Chocolate   180
    Peanut Butter   190

Teens, 1 pkg   225

Tempty, 1 pkg
    Chocolate   196
    Lemon   259

Tiger Tails   415
Twinkies   140

COFFEE CAKE, 1 cake

Almond
Sara Lee	1,350
Sara Lee Coffee Ring	1,100

Angel Food
Howard Johnson's	710

Apple
Morton	1,130
Sara Lee	1,175

Apple Cinnamon
Pillsbury	1,880

Apricot
Sara Lee	1,176

Banana
Sara Lee	1,440

Blueberry
Sara Lee Coffee Ring	1,080
Sara Lee Danish	1,175

Butter Pecan
Pillsbury	2,480

Butter Streusel
Sara Lee	1,395

Cherry
Sara Lee	1,050

Chocolate
Sara Lee	1,375

10

Chocolate, German
Morton	1,360
Sara Lee	1,230

Cinnamon Streusel
Pillsbury	2,000
Sara Lee	1,230

Coconut
Pepperidge Farm	1,940

Coffee Cake
Aunt Jemima	1,360

Crumb
Drake's	1,460

Lemon
Drake's	1,030

Maple Crunch
Sara Lee	1,157

Orange
Sara Lee	1,442

Pecan
Drake's	1,109
Morton	1,368
Sara Lee small	764
Sara Lee large	1,320

Raspberry
Sara Lee	1,090

Sour Cream
Pillsbury	2,160

COOKIES, 1 piece

Adelaide
  Pepperidge Farm 53
Almond
  Keebler 47
  Stella D'Oro 49
Almond Spice
  Keebler 50
Angel Puffs
  Stella D'Oro 17
Animal Crackers
  Keebler 12
  Nabisco 12
  Sunshine 10
Animal Crackers Iced
  Keebler 52
  Sunshine 26
Anise
  Stella D'Oro
    Anisette Sponge 50
    Anisette Toast 34
Apple
  Keebler 27
  Nabisco 48
Applesauce
  Sunshine 33
    Iced 104

Arrowroot
Nabisco   22
Sunshine   16

Assorted
Stella D'Oro
  Hostess   39
  Lady Stella   37

Bordeaux
Pepperidge Farm   37

Breakfast Treats
Stella D'Oro   100

Brown Edge
Nabisco   28

Brown Sugar
Nabisco   25
Pepperidge Farm   50

Brussels
Pepperidge Farm   57

Butter
Keebler   84
Nabisco   37
Pepperidge Farm   38
Sunshine   24

Capri
Pepperidge Farm   85

Cashew
Nabisco   57

Chessman
Pepperidge Farm   43

Chinese Dessert
Stella D'Oro   170
Chocolate
Keebler
Bavarian Fudge   80
Nut Fudge   31
Pecan Fudge   66
Melody   31
Nabisco
Wafers   28
Snaps   18
Pepperidge Farm   48
Sunshine   13
Chocolate Almond
Nabisco   55
Chocolate Brownies
Pepperidge Farm   57
Chocolate Chip
Chips Ahoy   50
Estee   30
Keebler   44
Old Fashioned   80
Rich 'N Chips   73
Townhouse   49
Nabisco   51
Family Favorite   33
Snaps   21
Pepperidge Farm   52
Sunshine   37
Chip-A-Roos   63

Chocolate Chip Coconut
Keebler	80
Nabisco	76
Sunshine	76

Chocolate Strawberry Wafers
Estee	90

Cinnamon
Sunshine	20

Cinnamon Almond
Nabisco	53

Cinnamon Sugar
Fun Days	48
Pepperidge Farm	52

Coconut
Keebler	61
Old Fashioned	83
Strip	37
Nabisco	16
Stella D'Oro	47
Sunshine	47

Coconut, Iced
Keebler Crunchies	70

Coconut Chocolate
Pepperidge Farm	83

Creme Sandwiches
Butterscotch
Keebler	85

Chocolate
Keebler Dutch	95

Keebler Opera	85
Oreo grocery	50
Oreo individual	40
Chocolate fudge	
Cookie Mates	53
Keebler	97
Sunshine	74
Coconut	
Nabisco	53
Sunshine	51
Wise Coco	39
Lemon	
Keebler	85
Swiss	
Nabisco	43
Vanilla	
Cameo	68
Cookie Mates	52
Keebler	82
French	95
Opera	85
Sunshine	79
Vienna Fingers	69
Wise	38
Crescents	
Nabisco	34
Cup Custard	
Sunshine	70
Danish Wedding	
Keebler	31

10

Date Nut
Pepperidge Farm   53
Sunshine   82

Devil's Food
Keebler   64
Nabisco   58
Sunshine   55

Dixie Vanilla
Sunshine   60

Egg Biscuits
Stella D'Oro   37
    Anise   135
    Egg Jumbo   43
    Rum and Brandy   135
    Sugared   135
    Vanilla   130

Figs
Nabisco Fig Newtons   59
Frito-Lay   189
Keebler   71
Sunshine   42

Fruit
Stella D'Oro   67
Sunshine Golden Fruit   61

Fruit, Iced
Nabisco   70

Fudge
Keebler
    Sticks   42

Strips | 57
Pepperidge Farm | 58

Gingerbread
Pepperidge Farm | 33

Gingerbread, Iced
Keebler | 130

Ginger Snaps
Keebler | 39
Nabisco | 30
Sunshine
  small | 14
  large | 32

Golden Bars
Stella D'Oro | 110

Graham Crackers
Keebler
  Honey | 17
  Thin | 17
  Very Thin | 14
Nabisco | 30
  Honey Maid | 30
Sunshine | 17
  Sugar Honey | 30

Graham Crackers, chocolate covered
Keebler | 44
Milco | 91
Nabisco | 55
  Fancy Dip | 68
Pantry | 62
Robena | 72

Kichel
Stella D'Oro 64
Lady Joan
Sunshine 42
Sunshine Iced 47
LaLanne
Sunshine 15
Lemon
Keebler 83
Nabisco 17
Sunshine 76
  Lemon Coolers 29
Lemon Nut
Pepperidge Farm 58
Lido
Pepperidge Farm 95
Love Cookies
Stella D'Oro 110
Macaroons
Sunshine 85
  Butter 39
  Coconut 81
Bake Shop 87
Nabisco 71
Mandel Toast
Stella D'Oro 54
Margherite
Stella D'Oro 73
Marigold Sandwich
Keebler 91

Marshmallow
Chocolate covered
Keebler
Dainties	68
Galaxies	82
Treasures	83
Tulips	83

Coconut
Nabisco	54
Sunshine	70

Iced
Sunshine
Frosted Cakes	68
Nut Sundae	74

Mallomars	60

Nabisco
Puffs	94
Twirls	133
Pinwheels	139

Sunshine
Puffs	63
Kings	135

Sandwich
Keebler	81
Nabisco	32

Sprinkles
Sunshine	71

Milano
Pepperidge Farm	63
Mint	70

10

Molasses Crisps
Pepperidge Farm   30
Molasses and Spice
Sunshine   67
Nassau
Pepperidge Farm   75
Oatmeal
Keebler   78
Nabisco
  Family Favorite   24
  Home Style   60
Sunshine   63
Oatmeal Almond
Pepperidge Farm   53
Oatmeal, Iced
Keebler   82
Oatmeal Marmalade
Pepperidge Farm   53
Oatmeal Peanut Butter
Sunshine   79
Oatmeal Raisin
Bake Shop   76
Nabisco   77
Pepperidge Farm   54
Orleans
Pepperidge Farm   33
Peanut
Pepperidge Farm   47
Sunshine   33

10

Raisin Bran
Pepperidge Farm   53

Shortbread
Keebler   27
Lorna Doone   38
Pepperidge Farm   65
Scottie   39

Shortbread with Cashews
Nabisco   50

Shortbread, Chocolate-covered
Nabisco   50

Shortbread with Coconut   65

Shortbread, Iced   58

Shortbread Pecans
Keebler   77
Nabisco   77

St. Moritz
Pepperidge Farm   47

Sorrento
Stella D'Oro   57

Sprinkles
Sunshine   57

Sugar
Eton   50
Keebler
  Giant   70
  Old Fashioned   81
Nabisco   17
Pepperidge Farm   53

Vanilla
  Keebler 19
  Nabisco
    Snaps 13
    Wafers 18
  Sunshine 15
Vanilla Thins
  Estee 25
Vienna Finger Sandwich
  Sunshine 71
Yum Yums
  Sunshine 83
Zanzibar
  Pepperidge Farm 37

PASTRY, FROZEN, MIXES, AND TOASTER, 1 piece unless noted

Dessert mixes
  Pillsbury Appleasy 160
Donuts
  Morton
    Bavarian Creme 180
    Boston Creme 205

Chocolate	150
Glazed	150
Jelly	180
Mini	120
Town House Cinnamon	210
Dumplings, apple	
Pepperidge Farm	280
Strudel, apple	
Pepperidge Farm, 1 oz	85
Tarts	
Kellogg's Pop Tarts	210
Pepperidge Farm	
Apple	280
Blueberry	285
Cherry	280
Lemon	310
Raspberry	320
Popovers (Flako)	166
Turnovers	
Pepperidge Farm	320
Pillsbury	180

PIES, FROZEN, 1 whole pie

Apple	
Banquet	1,440

Morton	1,740
Mini	590
Mrs. Smith's	1,768
Natural	2,881
Dutch	1,860
Tart	1,495

Banana Cream

Banquet	1,032
Morton	1,020
Mini	230
Mrs. Smith's	1,290
Light	1,320

Blueberry

Banquet	1,523
Morton	1,680
Mini	580
Mrs. Smith's	1,740
Natural	2,040

Boston Cream

| *Mrs. Smith's* | 1,980 |

Cherry

Banquet	1,360
Morton	1,805
Mini	591
Mrs. Smith's	1,860
Natural	2,040

Chocolate

| *Mrs. Smith's* | 1,500 |
| *Royal Dutch* | 2,040 |

Chocolate Cream
Banquet	1,060
Morton	1,200
Mini	260
Mrs. Smith's	1,470

Coconut
Mrs. Smith's	1,380

Coconut Cream
Banquet	1,040
Morton	1,140
Mini	260
Mrs. Smith's	1,380

Coconut Custard
Banquet	1,220
Morton	
Mini	370
Mrs. Smith's	1,590

Custard
Banquet	1,240

Devil Cream
Royal	2,280
Mrs. Smith's	1,470

Lemon
Mrs. Smith's	2,040
Royal	2,080

Lemon Cream
Banquet	1,000
Morton	1,000
Mini	240
Mrs. Smith's	1,350

10

Lemon Crunch
  Mrs. Smith's   2,480
Lemon Meringue
  Mrs. Smith's   1,560
Lemon Yogurt
  Mrs. Smith's   1,200
Mince
  Morton   1,860
    Mini   590
  Mrs. Smith's   2,010
Mincemeat
  Banquet   1,520
Neapolitan Cream
  Morton   1,140
  Mrs. Smith's   1,440
Nesselrode
  Royal   2,000
Peach
  Banquet   1,320
  Morton   1,680
    Mini   560
  Mrs. Smith's   1,800
    Natural   1,980
Pecan
  Morton
    Mini   580
  Mrs. Smith's   2,589
Pineapple
  Mrs. Smith's   1,800

Pineapple-Cheese
Mrs. Smith's	1,580

Pumpkin
Banquet	1,230
Morton	1,380
Mini	430
Mrs. Smith's	1,440

Raisin
Mrs. Smith's	1,890

Spumoni
Royal	2,120

Strawberry Cream
Banquet	1,020
Morton	1,080
Mrs. Smith's	1,320

Strawberry and Rhubarb
Mrs. Smith's	1,890
Natural	1,920

Strawberry-Yogurt
Mrs. Smith's	1,220

Pie Mixes, 1 whole pie

Betty Crocker Boston Cream	2,080
Pillsbury	
Chocolate Cream	2,460
Lemon Chiffon	1,980
Vanilla	2,340

10

Pie Crusts and Shells, 1 piece

Pastry Sheets	
Pepperidge Farm	570
Pastry Shells	
Pepperidge Farm	240
Stella D'Oro	146
Pie Crusts	
Betty Crocker	1,920
Stick	960
Flako	1,560
Pillsbury	1,740
Pie Shells	
Pepperidge Farm	521
shallow	440
with top	760
Stella D'Oro	240
Tart Shells	
Pepperidge Farm	88

Pie Fillings, 1 whole can unless noted

Apple	
Wilderness	660
Apricot	
Wilderness	720
Banana Cream	
Jell-O	660

Blueberry
Wilderness   660
Cherry
Wilderness   650
Lemon
Jell-O   1,080
Royal, 1 cup   310
Wilderness   840
Lime
Royal, 1 cup   310
Mince
Wilderness   840
Mincemeat
None Such, 1 cup   660
Peach
Wilderness   655
Pumpkin
Libby's, 1 cup   205
Stokely-Van Camp, 1 cup   370
Raisin
Wilderness   720
Strawberry
Wilderness   710

10
SMALL PASTRY PIES, 1 piece

Apple
Stella D'Oro 90
Hostess 400
Tastykake 350
Tastykake French 400
Blueberry
Hostess 365
Cherry
Hostess 420
Tastykake 380
Fig
Stella D'Oro 100
Guava
Stella D'Oro 125
Lemon
Hostess 420
Tastykake 355
Peach/Apricot
Stella D'Oro 90
Pecan
Frito-Lay 345
Prune
Stella D'Oro 92
Puff Pastry
Durkee
Beef 47

Cheese	59
Chicken	49
Chicken liver	48
Shrimp	44

PUDDINGS, MIXES AND CANNED, ½ cup, unless noted

Banana

Ann Page	250
Del Monte	180
Shak-A-Pudd'n	165
Royal	164

Banana Cream

Jell-O	175
My-T-Fine	175

Bavarian Cream

My-T-Fine	176

Butter Pecan

My-T-Fine	175

Butterscotch

Ann Page	190
Instant	170
Del Monte	175

D-Zerta	25
Foremost	175
Jell-O	172
My-T-Fine	170
Royal	190
Sego	250

Caramel Nut
Royal	195

Cherry
Whip 'n Chill	139

Cherry-Plum
Junket	135

Chocolate
Ann Page	180
Betty Crocker	180
Bounty	174
Dannon	150
Del Monte	250
D-Zerta	20
Foremost	175
Jell-O	175
Instant	190
My-T-Fine	185
Royal	190
Dark 'N Sweet	200
Sego	250
Shak-A-Pudd'n	200
Whip 'n Chill	145

Chocolate Almond
My-T-Fine	196

Chocolate Fudge
Betty Crocker	180
Del Monte	190
Foremost	175
Jell-O	175
Instant	191
My-T-Fine	190
Sego	250
Whip 'n Chill	139

Chocolate Malt
Shak-A-Pudd'n	200

Chocolate Marshmallow
Sego	250

Coconut
Ann Page	
Cream	190
Toasted	170
Jell-O	175
Instant	190
Royal	185

Currant-Raspberry
Junket	135

Custard
Ann Page	150
Jell-O	165
My-T-Fine	
Caramel	145
Vanilla	156
Rice-A-Roni	120
Royal	145

Indian
  B & M 150
Lemon
  Ann Page 150
    Instant 180
  Bounty 196
  Foremost 197
  Jell-O 178
    Instant 179
  My-T-Fine 180
  Royal 180
  Whip 'n Chill 135
Lemon Chiffon
  Jell-O 144
Mocha Nut
  Royal 190
Pineapple Cream
  Jell-O 165
    Instant 179
Pistachio
  Ann Page 180
  Royal 180
Plum
  Crosse & Blackwell 255
  R & R 300
Rice
  Betty Crocker 150
  Bounty 195
Strawberry
  Junket 135

Sego	250
Shak-A-Pudd'n	165
Whip 'n Chill	135

CHAPTER 11
Jellies, Syrups, Toppings and Spreads

DESSERT TOPPINGS, 1 Tbsp

Black Cherry
  No-Cal   0
Black Raspberry
  No-Cal   0
Butterscotch
  Hershey's   55
  Kraft   60
  Smucker's   69
Caramel
  Kraft
    chocolate   56

vanilla	57
Smucker's	69
peanut butter	75
Cherry	
Smucker's	65
Chocolate	
Bosco	50
Hershey's	45
Kraft	50
No-Cal	6
Smucker's	65
Tillie Lewis	16
Chocolate Fudge	
Hershey's	45
Kraft	70
Smucker's	65
Swiss	72
Chocolate Mint	
Hershey's	61
Smucker's	67
Chocolate Peanut Butter	
Hershey's	60
Coffee	
No-Cal	6
Cola	
No-Cal	0
Cream, whipped	
Reddi-Whip	8
Top-Whip	7

Grape
No-Cal   0
Hard Sauce
Crosse & Blackwell   64
Marshmallow
Kraft   35
Pecans in Syrup
Kraft   82
Smucker's   65
Pineapple
Kraft   50
Smucker's   62
Strawberry
Kraft   45
No-Cal   0
Smucker's   60
Walnut
Kraft   88
Walnuts in Syrup
Smucker's   65
Whip, non-dairy
Cool Whip   14
D-Zerta   8
Dream Whip   10
Kraft   9
Lucky Whip   11
Pet   16
Reddi-Whip   9

FROSTINGS, 1 can

Betty Crocker
Chocolate Fudge	1920
Coconut Pecan	1310
White, creamy	1920
White, fluffy *Lite*	720
All other flavors	1800

Pillsbury
Coconut Pecan	1800
White, fluffy	840
All other flavors	2040

GELATIN, ½ cup

Borden's
Cherry	80
Fruit Cocktail	109
Mandarin Orange	89
Perfection	81
Pineapple-papaya	78
Pineapple-raspberry	77
Strawberry	75

Jell-O
1-2-3	81
Best	77
Knox unflavored, dry, 1 envelope	28
Royal	80

JELLIES AND BUTTERS, 1 Tbsp

Apple Butter
Bama	31
Smucker's	
Cider	39
Spiced	39
Peach	45
Ma Brown	32
Musselman's	33

Jams
Ann Page	51
Bama	51
Diet Delight	22
Kraft	49
S & W	10
Smucker's	54
Slenderella	24
artificially sweetened	1

Jellies

Ann Page	54
Bama	51
Crosse & Blackwell	51
Diet Delight	21
Home Brands	54
Kraft	48
Low Calorie	22
Ma Brown	49
Musselman's	53
S & W	12
Smucker's	51
Slenderella	24
Single Service	50
Welch's	50

Marmalade

Ann Page	54
Bama	54
Kraft	54
Low Calorie	25
S & W	11
Smucker's	49
Slenderella	24

Preserves

Ann Page	54
Bama	51
Crosse & Blackwell	59
Empress	54
Home Brands	54
Kraft	48

Low Calorie	25
Regular	55
Ma Brown	51
S & W	11
Smucker's	54
Welch's	54
Spreads	
Smucker's	24
Tillie Lewis	12

SPREADS, 1 Tbsp

Anchovy Paste	
Crosse & Blackwell	20
Chicken	
Swanson	35
Underwood	32
Chicken Salad	
Carnation	31
Corned Beef	
Underwood	28
Ham	
Carnation	26
Hormel	35
Libby's	100
Underwood	48

11

Liverwurst
Underwood   46
Peanut Butter
Ann Page   105
Bama   100
   and jelly   82
Datetree   93
Home Brands   100
Jif   93
Kitchen King   95
Peter Pan   94
Planters   95
Roberts   93
Skippy   95
Smucker's   95
   Goober Grape   63
Sultana   101
Potted Meat
Libby's   140
Roast Beef
Underwood   29
Sandwich Spread
Best Foods   60
Hellman's   58
Mrs. Filbert's   53
Nu Made   51
Oscar Mayer   33
Spam
Hormel   40

Tuna
  Carnation   26
Turkey Salad
  Carnation   27

SUGAR, SYRUPS, SWEETENERS AND HONEY

Honey, 1 Tbsp   64
  1 cup   1,031
Sugar, 1 cup
  Brown
    loosely packed   540
    firmly packed   820
  Maple   790
  Powdered   460
    sifted   385
  White, granulated   770
    1 Tbsp   45
Sweeteners, Sugar Substitutes
  Dia-Mel Sugar-Like, 1 gram pkt   3
  Dia-Mel Sweet'n-it Liquid   0
  Featherweight Sug'r Like, 1 tsp   2
  Pillsbury Sprinkle Sweet, 1 tsp   2

11

Pillsbury Sweet 10	0
Sweet'n Low, 1 gram pkt	3½
Weight Watchers Sweet'ner, 1 gram pkt	3
Whitlock Suprose, 1 gram pkt	4
Syrup, 1 Tbsp	
Aunt Jemima	53
Cary's Diet	10
Cary's Maple	60
Diet Delight	15
Golden Griddle	50
Karo	60
Corn	58
Maple	54
Log Cabin	
Buttered	52
Country Kitchen	53
Maple	46
Maple-Honey	55
Mrs. Butterworth's	54
S & W	12
Tillie Lewis	14
Molasses	
dark	45
light	50
Sorghum	55

CHAPTER 12

Candies, Ice Cream and Nuts

CANDY, 1 oz

12

Jellied Candy

Dots	100
Jujubes	50
Jujyfruits	94
Mason	99
Quaker City	93
Red Hot Dollars	94

Licorice

Black Crows	101
Diamond Drops	98
Good & Plenty	99
Heide Pastilles	96
Switzer	97

Lifesavers, 1 piece   7

Malted Milk

Walter Johnson	131

Mars   126

Marshmallows

Campfire	100
Curtiss	97
Kraft	96
Jet Puff	125
Macaroon	110

Milky Way   119

Mints

Kraft	105
Richardson	110

Mints, chocolate-coated

Mason	203

GUM, 1 piece

Adams	9
Beeman	10
Beech-Nut	9
Beechies	6
Black Jack	9
Bubble Yum	25
Bubblicious	24
Care Free	8
Chiclets	6
Clorets	6
Clove	5
Dentyne	5
Estee	3
Freshen-Up	9
Fruit Stripe	9
Orbit	8
Trident	5
Wrigley's	10

ICE CREAM, 1 cup (½ pint)

Black Raspberry
   Breyer's   264
Black Walnut
   Meadow Gold   329
Butter Almond
   Sealtest   326
Butter Almond and Chocolate
   Breyer's   318
Butter Brickle
   Sealtest   299
Butter Pecan
   Meadow Gold   300
   Sealtest   322
Butterscotch Pecan
   Breyer's   302
Caramel Pecan
   Breyer's   320
Cherry
   Sealtest   276
Cherry-Vanilla
   Breyer's   280
   Meadow Gold   280
   Sealtest   265
Chocolate
   Borden's   255
   Breyer's   314

Howard Johnson's	414
Meadow Gold	281
Sealtest	254
Swift's	242
Vanilla	
Bordens	246
Breyer's	299
Carnation	250
Howard Johnson's	500
Meadow Gold	280
Sealtest	289
Swift's	267
Sealtest	280
Vanilla-Fudge	
Breyer's	300
Vanilla-Raspberry	
Sealtest	279

Ice Milk, 1 cup   200

Sherbet, 1 cup   260

Ice Cream Bars, 1

Bi-sicle	110
Creamsicle	78
Dreamsicle	70
Dreamstick	180
Drumstick	183
Fudgesicle	100
Good Humor	
Almond	218
Chocolate	222
Ice	50
Chocolate-covered vanilla	169
Whammy	105
Popsicle	72
Sealtest	
Orange Cream	71
Orange Treat	89

Ice Cream Cones and Cups, 1 item

Comet	
cone	19
cone, rolled sugar	35
cup	20

12

Take-Out Ice Cream, 1 item

Baskin Robbins

Banana Daiquiri Ice	129
Butter Pecan	195
Chocolate Fudge	229
Chocolate Mint	189
Jamoca	182
Mango Sherbert	132
Peach	165
Rocky Road	205
Strawberry	168
Vanilla	217

Bridgeman's

Plain cone	170
Sugar cone	200

Dairy Queen

Banana Split	540
Cone	
large	340
medium	230
small	110
Float	330
Freeze	520
Malt	
large	840
medium	600
small	340
Parfait	460
Sandwich	140

Sundae
large	400
medium	300
small	170

Friendly's
Fribble
chocolate	470
vanilla	420

Sundae
vanilla fudge	420
vanilla strawberry	340

NUTS AND SEEDS, 1 oz

Almonds
Blue Diamond	179
Franklin	154
Granny Goose	155
Planters	170

Cashews
A & P	170
Frito-Lay	170
Franklin	145
Granny Goose	170
Planters	170
Skippy	163

Filberts
Franklin   164
Mixed
A & P   190
Excel   190
Franklin   160
   with peanuts   156
Granny Goose   168
Planters   180
   with peanuts   185
Skippy   172
Peanuts
A & P   180
   in shell   170
Excel   180
Frito-Lay   175
   in shell   160
   Spanish   170
Granny Goose   168
Planters   170
   Spanish, dry roasted   162
   Peanut Crisps   150
Skippy   165
Tavern Nuts   171
Pecans
A & P   200
Granny Goose   203
Planters   190
Pistachios
Frito-Lay   174

CHAPTER 13

Fast Foods and Snacks

CHIPS, PUFFS, CRISPS, ETC.

1 oz unless noted

Salted	121
Sesame	119
Whole wheat	122
Taco Chips	
Old London	127
Tortilla Chips	
Doritos	
Nachos	137
Tacos	142
Granny Goose	144
Planters	
Nachos	128
Tacos	132
Wheat Chips	
Bakon Snacks	147

PIZZA, FROZEN, 1 whole
pizza unless noted

Beef and Cheese	
El Chico	
with enchilada	1,010
with taco	990
Bacon	
Tostino's	704

Cheese
Buitoni	276
Celeste	473
large	1,280
Sicilian	1,395
with mushroom, small	459
with mushroom, large	1,205
Chef Boy-Ar-Dee	798
small	160
Jeno's	840
Deluxe	1,470
Junior	165
Mix	838
Kraft	822
Pee Wee	170
Lambrecht	909
La Pizzeria	1,230
Lean Cuisine	170
Roman	891
Stouffer's	330
Tostino's	882

Cheese and Refried Beans
El Chico	902

Cheese and Chili
El Chico	1,039

Combinations
Celeste	600
large	1,480
Jeno's Deluxe	1,667

La Pizzeria	830
large	1,529
Stouffer's	789
Tostino's	1,683
Classic	1,675
Hamburger	
Jeno's	888
Tostino's	910
Crisp	955
Open Face	
Buitoni	250
Pepperoni	
Celeste	540
large	1,438
Chef Boy-Ar-Dee	175
Jeno's	901
La Pizzeria	1,322
Roman	889
Stouffer's	800
Tostino's	923
Crisp	960
Classic	1,792
Classic with mushrooms	1,497
Rolls	
Jeno's	
Cheeseburger	268
Pepperoni	262
Sausage	259
Shrimp	214

Sausage

Celeste	561
large	1,500
Jeno's	899
Deluxe	1,495
Mix	1,058
Kraft	1,000
Pee Wee	190
Lambrecht	1,005
La Pizzeria	860
large	1,515
Roman	233
Tostino's	938
Crisp	981
Classic	1,799

POPCORN AND PRETZELS

Popcorn, 1 cup

Jiffy Pop	31
Jolly Time	31
King Korn	
Cheese	40
Seasoned	42
Pops-Rite	38

Presto-Pop	37
3 Minute	38
TNT	52
Wise	43
Cheese-flavored	49
Wonder	45
Pretzels, 1 piece	
Bachman	
B's	8
Beer	55
Medium	20
Teeny	11
Thin	18
Old London	5
Nabisco Mister Salty	
Dutch	51
3-Ring	12
Veri-Thin	20
Pretzelettes	6
Sunshine	19

FAST FOODS

Arby's	
Beef and Cheese Sandwich	450
Club Sandwich	560

Ham and Cheese Sandwich	380
Junior Roast Beef Sandwich	220
Roast Beef Sandwich	350
Super Roast Beef Sandwich	620
Swiss King Sandwich	660
Turkey Deluxe Sandwich	510
Turkey Sandwich	410

Arthur Treacher's

Chicken	271
Chicken Sandwich	265
Chips	243
Chowder	66
Cole Slaw	144
Fish	241
Fish Sandwich	282
Krunch Pup	358
Lemon Luvs	324
Shrimp	380

Brazier (Dairy Queen)

Hamburger	260
Cheeseburger	320
Big Brazier	460
Big Brazier with Cheese	550
Big Brazier with Lettuce and Tomato	470
Super Brazier (The Half-Pounder)	780
Hot Dog	270
Hot Dog with Chili	330
Hot Dog with Cheese	330
Fish Sandwich	400
Fish Sandwich with Cheese	440

French Fries	200
French Fries, large	320
Onion Rings	300

Burger Chef

Chocolate Shake	310
Big Chef	542
Cheeseburger	304
Double Cheeseburger	434
Double Hamburger	325
French Fries	187
Hamburger	258
Mariner Platter	680
Rancher Platter	640
Shake	326
Skipper's Treat	604
Super Chef	600

Burger King

Whopper	650
Double Beef *Whopper*	850
Whopper with Cheese	760
Double Beef *Whopper* with Cheese	970
Whopper Junior	360
Whopper Junior with Cheese	420
Whopper Junior with Double Meat	490
Whopper Junior Double Meat with Cheese	550
Hamburger	310
Hamburger with Cheese	360
Double Meat Hamburger	440
Double Meat Hamburger with Cheese	540

Steak Sandwich	600
Whaler	660
Whaler with Cheese	770
Onion Rings, large	330
Onion Rings, regular	230
French Fries, large bag	360
French Fries, regular bag	240
Chocolate Milkshake	380
Vanilla Milkshake	360
Apple Pie	240

Carl's Jr.

Famous Star Hamburger	480
Super Star Hamburger	660
Old Time Star Hamburger	440
Happy Star Hamburger	290
Steak Sandwich	630
California Roast Beef Sandwich	380
Fish Fillet Sandwich	550
Original Hot Dog	340
Chili Dog	360
Chili Cheese Dog	400
American Cheese	40
Salad with Condiments 11 oz	170
Dressing, 2 oz	
Blue Cheese	200
Thousand Island	190
Lo-Cal Italian	48
French Fries	220
Apple Turnover	330

Carrot Cake	380
Shake	310
Soft Drinks	200

Church's Fried Chicken, 1 piece, boned

| Dark | 305 |
| White | 327 |

Dunkin' Donuts

Cake and Chocolate Cake Donuts	
rings, sticks, crullers, etc.	240
Yeast-raised Donuts	160
Glazed Yeast-Raised Donuts	168
Fancies	
coffee rolls, danish, etc.	215
Fancies with Filling and Topping	260
Munchkins, Yeast-raised	26
Munchkins, Cake and Chocolate Cake	66
Munchkins with Filling and Topping	79

Gino's

Apple Pie	238
Cheeseburger	300
Cheese Hero	738
Cheese Sirloiner	532
Coke	117
Fish Platter	650
Fish Sandwich	450
French Fries	156
Giant	569
Hamburger	254
Hero	647
Hot Chocolate	90

Hardees

Apple Turnover	282
Big Twin	447
Cheeseburger	335
Deluxe	675
Double Cheeseburger	495
Fish Sandwich	468
French Fries, large	381
French Fries, small	239
Hamburger	305
Hot Dog	346
Milkshake	391
Roast Beef Sandwich	390

Jack-in-the-Box

Apple Turnover	411
Breakfast Jack	301
Cheeseburger	
Deluxe	310
Jumbo Jack	628
Double Cheese Omelet	423
French Fries	270
French Toast	537
Hamburger	
Bonus Jack	461
Deluxe	260
Jumbo Jack	551
Ham and Cheese Omelet	425
Jack Burrito	448
Jack Steak	428
Lemon Turnover	446

Moby Jack	455
Onion Rings	351
Pancakes	626
Ranchero Omelet	414
Scrambled Eggs	719
Shakes, Chocolate	365
Strawberry	380
Vanilla	342
Taco	189
Taco Super	285

Kentucky Fried Chicken

Chicken Dinner
   (3 pieces chicken, potatoes, cole slaw, roll)

| Original Recipe Dinner | 830 |
| Extra Crispy Dinner | 950 |

Individual Pieces

Wing	151
Drumstick	136
Keel	253
Rib	242
Thigh	276

Long John Silver's

Breaded Clams	465
Breaded Oysters	460
Chicken planks	458
Cole Slaw	138
Corn on the Cob	174
Fish with Batter, 2 pieces	318
Fries	375

Hush Puppies	153
Ocean Scallops	257
Peg Leg	514
Shrimp	268
Treasure Chest	467

McDonald's

Apple Pie	300
Big Mac	541
Cheeseburger	306
Cherry Pie	298
Chocolate Shake	364
Egg McMuffin	352
English Muffin, Buttered	186
Fillet O' Fish	402
French Fries	211
Hamburger	257
Hot Cakes, with Butter or Syrup	472
McDonaldland Cookies	294
Quarter-pounder	418
Quarter-pounder with Cheese	518
Sausage	184
Scrambled eggs	162
Shake, Strawberry	345
Shake, Vanilla	323

Pizza Hut, 1 slice, Thin

Standard

Cheese	180
Pepperoni	202
Pork and Mushroom	196

Super Supreme	266
Superstyle	
Cheese	213
Pepperoni	233
Pork and Mushroom	230
Supreme	216

Ponderosa, Entree

Chopped Beef	324
Double Deluxe	362
Extra-cut Prime Rib	409
Extra-cut Ribeye	358
Fillet of Sole	251
Fillet of Sole Sandwich	125
Junior Patty	98
Prime Rib	286
Ribeye	259
Ribeye/Shrimp	400
Shrimp	220
Steakhouse Deluxe	181
Strip Sirloin	277
Super Sirloin	383
T-Bone	374

Poppin' Fresh

Chef's Salad	800
Custard Pie, 1 slice	380
Dairy Salad	650
Dinner Salad	250
Doughboy Salad	530
Pumpkin Pie, 1 slice	390

13

Shrimp Salad	640
Tuna Salad	640

Steak 'N Shake

Steakburger	276
Steakburger with Cheese	352
Super Steakburger	375
Super Steakburger with Cheese	451
Triple Steakburger	474
Triple Steakburger with Cheese	625
Low Calorie Platter	293
Baked Ham Sandwich	451
Toasted Cheese Sandwich	250
Ham & Egg Sandwich	434
Egg Sandwich	275
French Fries	211
Chili and Oyster Crackers	337
Chili	402
Baked Beans	173
Lettuce and Tomato Salad with 1 oz Thousand Island Dressing	168
Chef Salad	313
Cottage Cheese	93
Apple Danish	391
Sundaes	
Strawberry	329
Hot Fudge Nut	530
Brownie Fudge	645
Apple Pie	407
Cherry Pie	334

Cheesecake	368
Brownie	259

Taco Bell

Bean Burrito	343
Beef Burrito	466
Beefy Tostada	291
Bellbeefer	221
Bellbeefer with Cheese	278
Burrito Supreme	457
Combination Burrito	404
Enchirito	454
Pintos Cheese	168
Taco	186
Tostada	179

Wendy's

Cheeseburger

Single cheese	580
Double cheese	800
Triple cheese	1,040
Chili	230
French Fries	330
Frosty	390

Hamburger

Single	470
Double	670
Triple	850

White Castle

Cheeseburger	185
Fish	192

13

French Fries   225
Hamburger   160

Zantiago
Burrito   345
Enchirito   391
Frijoles   231
Taco   146
Tostada   206

CHAPTER 14

Home Cooked, Restaurant and Frozen

HOME COOKED AND RESTAURANT DISHES,
1 average portion unless noted

Abalone with mushrooms	526
Abalone with oyster sauce	283
Abalone steaks	215
Aioli sauce, 1 Tbsp	125
Almond tarts, each	70
Alu Bhaji	130

Ambrosia	126
Ambrosia salad	542
Anchovy butter, 1 Tbsp	127
Angel Food Cake	120
Apples, baked	225
Apples, stuffed	265
Apple Brown Betty	547
Apples, candied	355
Apple Caramel	488
Apple cinnamon rings	180
Apple curried rings	155
Apple fried rings	165
Apple, pickled, 1 apple	50
Applesauce	225
Apple turnovers	400
Apricot, Brown Betty	498
Armenian style mussels, stuffed with rice, currants and piñon nuts	528
Arroz con Pollo	655
Artichoke, boiled	146
Artichoke hearts, marinated	75
Artichokes, Jerusalem boiled	163
Artichoke moutarde	374
Artichoke, Provencal-style, braised	127
Artichoke vinaigrette	446
Asparagus, buttered	90
Asparagus, Chinese-style	150
Asparagus Divan, 4 spears	375
Asparagus vinaigrette	170

Beef and Asparagus   929
   and Bean Curd   682
   and Bean Sprouts   646
   and Broccoli   585
   Congee   896
   Consommé, 1 cup   33
   Fondue Bourguignonne   479
   and Green Pepper   444
   Lo Mein   1,042
   and Mushrooms   435
   and Noodles in Brown Bean Sauce   685
   and Oyster Sauce   689
   with Pea Pods and Water Chestnuts   648
   and Mushroom Pirog   720
   Picadillo   400
Beef Brisket   530
Beef Heart, stuffed   475
Beef Kidneys, braised   275
Beef Roasts
   Pot-au-feu   555
   Pot Roast   600
   Pot Roast, French-style   715
   Pot Roast, German-style   650
   Sauerbraten   569
   Yankee Pot Roast   746
Beef Short Ribs   485
Beef Steak
   Bracioulini   423
   Chicken-fried   935
   Chinese-style   345

Diane	600
Diavolo	621
en croute	685
Esterhazy	977
Flank, broiled	380
Florentine	460
Kew	475
London Broil	380
alla pizzaiola	668
au poivre	525
au poivre flamée	492
swiss	655
tartare	347
Beef Stew	
Bourguignonne	639
Carbonnade Flamande	639
with Dumplings	874
Hungarian Goulash	388
Indonesian Spiced	738
Old-fashioned	695
Oxtail	465
Steak and Kidney Pie	949
Stroganoff	427
Beef Sukiyaki	185
Beef Teriyaki	300
Beef Tongue	
pickled	389
jellied	310
baked	112
boiled	112

14

Beets

harvard in sour cream	170
in horseradish	120
pickled, 1 beet	10
Beignet d 'Aubergines, 4 oz	200
Beurre Manié, 1 Tbsp	98
Bhendi Bhaji	85
Bernaise Sauce, 1 Tbsp	46
Billi-Bi	222
Biscuit Tortoni	284
Biscuit, Baking Powder, 1 piece	83
Black Bean dip, 1 Tbsp	36
Black-eyed peas, Southern-style	550
Black forest cake	758
Blancmange	162
Blanquette de Veau	699
Blini, 1 piece	87
with butter	184
with caviar	204
Blintzes, cheese, 1 piece	177
Blood Sausage, 6 oz	708
Blueberry muffins	133
Blueberry waffles	259
Bocconcini	524
Bordelaise sauce, 1 Tbsp	23
Borscht	400
Boston Baked beans	534
Boston Brown Bread, 1 slice	86
Bougatsa, 1 piece	401
Bouillabaisse	600

Bourek, 1 piece	98
Brains with Almonds	653
braised	338
with sherry	570
Brandied Peaches, 1 peach	65
Bratwurst, grilled, 6 oz	500
Bratwurst, sauteed, 6 oz	563
Brandy Alexander pie	680
Brandy sauce, 1 Tbsp	44
hard, 1 Tbsp	115
Brandy snaps, 1 piece	98
Brazilian Black Beans	376
Bread sauce, 1 Tbsp	18
Brioche	201
Broccoli amandine	279
Broccoli with Parmesan	105
Brownie, 1 piece	160
Buche de Noel	684
Buffalo Steak, broiled	400
Bulgar, pilaf	290
plain	277
Buttermilk Biscuits, 1 piece	88
Buttermilk salad dressing, 1 Tbsp	9
Butterscotch Brownie, 1 piece	156
Butterscotch Sauce, 1 Tbsp	71
Burrito with Beans	321
with Chili	251
with Beef and Beans	335
Bytky	631

Cabbage

Austrian	227
Baked	106
Colcannon	144
Creole	133
Flemish Red, with Apples	268
Pennsylvania Dutch	155
Pickled, 1 cup	200
Polish	400
Rolls Stuffed with Lamb	372
Sweet and Sour	150
Cacciucco	414
Cacik	100
Caesar salad	299

Cake

Applesauce	205
Cheesecake	424
Cheesecake, Italian style	520
Chocolate	230
Cinnamon and Coffee	135
Coconut cream	240
Devil's food	240
Lemon Chiffon	300
Light Fruit	266
Genoese	120
Marble	195
Petits fours, 1 piece	251
Pineapple Upside-down	255
Rainbow	210
Sachertorte	362

Celeri Rémoulade, 4 oz	303
Celeriac, creamed	213
Ceviche	308
Champ	157
Champignon farci gratinée, 1 piece	135
Chantilly Sauce, 1 Tbsp	75
Chard, pureed	107
Char shu ding	300
Charlotte Russe	458
Chasseur Sauce, 1 Tbsp	31
Cheese Boreks	138
Cheese Dumplings, 1 piece	95
Cheese Fondue	1,000
Cheese straws, 10 pieces	283
Cheese sauce, 1 Tbsp	38
Cheese souffle	327
Cherries Jubilee	200
Chestnuts	
creamed	400
pureed	327
roasted, 6 oz	245
Chicken	
and Almonds	750
and Asparagus	510
Barbecued with Skin and Bones	405
Bhuna	219
and Black Bean Sauce	748
Burmese, in Peanut and Coconut Sauce	845
Cacciatore	468
and Cashews	750

Musallam	227
with Mushrooms	528
Pancake, Chinese-style	899
Parmigiana	510
Pizziola	290
Roumanian-style, with Apricots	468
Salad	423
with Snow peas	520
Stew	560
stuffed with rice and mushrooms	362
Sub Gum	638
Sweet and Sour	1,150
Tandoori	366
Teriyaki	878
Tetrazzini	878
Chinese-style, with vegetables	670
Velvet	742
Vino bianco	300
with walnuts	929
Yakitori	253
Zingara	500
and tomato salad	199
Chili	448
Chiles con Queso	327
Chiles Rellenos	442
Chiles de Frijoles	544
Chimichango	288
Chinese style	
Beef	343
Cabbage, quickfried	200

Cabbage, steamed	85
Cabbage, Sweet and Sour	200
Carp, Sweet and Sour	300
Mustard Sauce, 1 Tbsp	5
Egg roll	145
Fried eggs and Rice	324
Fried puffs, 1 piece	86
Fried rice	301
Pork with rice	277
Shrimp with ginger	274
Snow peas	115
Spareribs	565
Sweet and sour sauce, 1 Tbsp	15
Cucumber and soy sauce	62

Chocolate

Chiffon Cake, 1 slice	318
Chip Cookie, 1 piece	75
Eclairs	282
Mousse	316
Profiteroles, 1 piece	153
Sauce, 1 Tbsp	86
Hot Soufflé	339

Chinese fried puffs, 1 piece	86
Chopped Chicken liver, ½ cup	262
Chorizos, 1 link	147

Chutney, 1 Tbsp

Coconut	17
Green Tomato	25
Mango	63

Mint	10
Tomato	30
Clams	
Bisque	200
in Black Bean Sauce, Chinese-style, 1	39
Casino, 1 dozen	536
New England Pie	325
Origanata, 1 dozen	440
Red Sauce	301
White Sauce	142
Cockaleekie	95
Cocoa	175
Coconut Macaroon, 1 piece	57
Cod Kedgeree	333
Coleslaw and caraway salad	238
Court Bouillon	4
Couscous, Boiled	305
Beef	567
Chicken	653
Lamb	600
Coquilles Saint-Jacques	475
Cornbread, 1 slice	100
Corn Fritters	249
relish, 1 Tbsp	16
sticks, per stick	100
Corned beef and cabbage	600
Corned beef hash	400
Coulibiac	288
Crab	
Cakes, Maryland-style	257

Cocktail, ½ cup	92
Deviled	398
Legs, Alaska King	297
Louis	767
Meunière, 2	278
Mornay	513
Newburg Imperial	426
Cranberry Nut Bread, 1 slice	136
Cranberry Relish, 1 Tbsp	44
Cranberry sauce, 1 Tbsp	28
Cream Cheese Dip, with Bacon and Horseradish, 1 Tbsp	74
Cream Puff, 1 piece	251
Creme brulee	655
Creme Caramel	280
Crepes, au champignon, 1 piece	178
Crepes, au jambon gratinée, 1 piece	156
Crepes Suzette, 1 piece	208
Crispy Bass, Chinese-style	484
Croissant, 1 piece	90
Croque Madame	710
Croque Monsieur	710
Croquettes de crevette	263
Croquettes de volaille	493
Cucumber and yogurt sauce, 1 Tbsp	5
Crumpet, 1 piece	80
Cumberland sauce, 1 Tbsp	40
Curried	
Beef	415
Beef Triangles, 1 piece	154

Lamb	656
Lamb and dhal	870
Cold lobster	493
Shrimp	504
Custard, baked	162
Custard, floating island	253
Custard, rennet	107
Custard sauce	27
Danish pastry	144
Datenut bread, 1 slice	88
Dhal	229
Deviled Ham, 1 Tbsp	38
Diable sauce, 1 Tbsp	20
Dijonnaise sauce, 1 Tbsp	93
Dips, 1 Tbsp	
Black bean	37
Chili	18
Clam in Cream Cheese	75
Cream cheese, bacon and horseradish	71
Curry	40
Deviled clam	80
Taramasalata	102
Divinity, 1 piece	38
Dolma	225
Doughnut	
chocolate, 1 piece	175
jelly	147
old fashioned	135
Duck	
with Cherry sauce	400

Fried	281
Greek-style	195
Greek-style, stuffed	180
Ismir	246
Parmigiana	598
Pisto	135
Ratatouille	510
Stuffed with mushrooms and chickpeas	228
Stuffed with pilaf and raisins	188
Turkish	327
Egg Rolls, Chinese, 1 piece	145
Empanada, with beef	244
Empanada, with chicken	220
Enchilada	
Beef	299
Cheese	270
Chicken	330
Chorizo	267
Escalopes de veau cordon bleu	680
Escargot de bourgogne, 6 pieces	418
Escarole, sautéed	74
Esterhazy steak	994
Falafel	263
Fennel, braised	116
Fettuccine Alfredo	1,550
Fettuccine con Baccala	653
Figs, fresh stewed	195
Finnan Haddie	257
Fish balls, Chinese-style, 8 oz	319

Fish, Jade Chinese-style, 6 oz	547
Lemon Chinese-style, 8 oz	754
Fish mousse	286
Fish piquant en papillote	199
Fish soufflé	300
Flan	263
Flemish red cabbage and apples	248
Floating island	257
Florentines, 1 piece	118
Flounder fillet in black bean sauce	600
Fondue de Gruyère	478
Fragrant noodles with shrimp, Chinese-style	810
Franks in blankets, 1 piece	46
French-fried onion rings	165
French-fried potatoes	227
Frijoles fritos	325
Frijoles Mexicanos	194
Frikadeller	384
Fruit cake, light, 1 slice	264
Fudge, chocolate, 1 piece	78
Fudge Sauce, hot, 1 Tbsp	100
Garlic bread, 1 slice	88
Garlic sauce, 1 Tbsp	11
Gefilte fish	183
Giblet gravy, 1 Tbsp	16
Gingersnaps, 1 piece	97
Gingerbread, 1 slice	206
Gingerbread boys, 1 boy	132
Gnocchi, Cheese	410

Gumbo, shrimp	308
Haddock, Baked	300
Creamy smoked and potato casserole	425
Ham	
in aspic	600
fried with red eye gravy	400
loaf	427
Tetrazzini	590
Hamburger	
bacon	400
broiled	280
cheese	370
chili	285
Pizza	285
mushroom	270
Hash	310
Hawaiian spareribs	409
Herb Butter, 1 Tbsp	125
Herring	
and beets a la Russe	591
in dill sauce	188
in mustard sauce	150
in oatmeal	370
Pickled	217
Rollmops	239
Scandanavian salad	379
in sour cream	127
Hoagie, 1 roll	400
Hog Jowl and Black-Eyed Peas	351
Hollandaise sauce, 1 Tbsp	48

Horseradish cream sauce, 1 Tbsp	77
Horseradish, fresh, 1 Tbsp	5
Hot Chocolate	275
Hot Cross Bun, 1 piece	105
Huevos Rancheros, 1 egg	186
Humus with tahini, ½ cup	364
Hushpuppies, 1 piece	67
Indian Corn Fritters, 1 piece	50
Indian Pudding	371
Indian Rice Pilaf	395
Irish Soda Bread, 1 slice	114
Irish Stew	710
Japanese Salad	
autumn	150
cucumber	48
cucumber and fish	135
cucumber and seaweed	64
lotus root	87
Jelly, homemade, 1 Tbsp	45
Jelly Roll	187
Jhinga Bhajia, 1 piece	37
Jhinga Kari, 10-12 shrimp	609
Jhonnycake, 1 piece	98
Kasha, buckwheat	355
appel-almond	400
Katsudon	829
Kebabs, Indian lamb	231
Kedgeree	318
Keema curry	246
Keftedakia Marinata	410

Keftedes	248
Keftedes Avgolemono	200
Khiri Pachadi	122
Kibbeh	964
Kidneys, braised	289
Kielbasa, fried, 3 oz	350
Kissel	240
Knockwurst, sauteed, 6 oz	538
Korma curry	344
Koulebiaka	1,300
Kourabiedes, 1 piece	75
Kreplach, 1 piece	34
Kugelhupf, 1 slice	187
Ladyfingers, 1 piece	52
Lamb	
braised	490
breast	425
cassoulet	1,050
crown roast	270
dolma	232
kidneys in sour cream	485
riblets, barbecued	840
shanks	372
shish kebab	686
stew	403
Lancashire Hot Pot	552
Lasagne, with cheese	605
with meat	408
with meat balls	1,095
Lebkuchen, 1 piece	84

Moo goo gai pan	244
Mornay sauce, 1 Tbsp	33
Moules	
farcis provencale, 8–10 pieces	324
gratinées Normande, 8–10 pieces	285
Marseille, 8–10 pieces	450
salade de, 8–10 pieces	461
vinaigrette, 8–10 pieces	230
Moussaka	818
Mousse, Avocado	196
Chocolate	306
Fish	282
Mozzarella cheese, breaded and fried	231
Muffin, 1 piece	108
Bran	140
Corn	148
Raisin bran	162
Mushroom gravy, 1 Tbsp	26
Mushrooms	
creamed	200
in madeira	236
marinated	51
sauteed	187
Mushrooms with bamboo shoots	295
Mu shu pork, 2 pancakes	874
Mustard sauce, 1 Tbsp	41
Nachos, 1 piece	40
Nantua sauce, 1 Tbsp	24
Napoleons, 1 piece	402

Napolitos	100
New England boiled dinner	735
Nockerln	163
Noodles in brown bean sauce and pork	891
Noodles in oyster sauce	463
Normandy rock cornish game hen, 1 bird	700
Oatmeal Bread, 1 slice	120
Octopus Mediterranean	350
Okra, fried	175
Omelet	
with caviar, 1 egg	180
Greek, 1 egg	130
Lorraine, 1 egg	167
Lyonnaise, 1 egg	136
with mushroom and tomato, 1 egg	135
Onion frittata, 1 egg	200
Piperade, 1 egg	215
Soufflé, 1 egg	111
Spanish, 1 egg	127
Onion Rings, french-fried	184
Onions, baked, 1 piece	155
Onions, creamed	209
sautéed	150
stuffed	186
Oshi tashi	34
Osso buco	905
Oysters casino, 1 dozen	540
Oysters en Brochette	215
Oysters Rockefeller, 1 dozen	1,000

Oyster Sauce, 1 Tbsp	35
Paella	
with lobster	620
with sausage	630
Valenciana	548
Pakora (Indian fritters)	
Baigon	41
Gobhi	38
Mixed vegetable	54
Pancakes, 1 piece	
apple	95
blueberry	87
buckwheat	82
buttermilk	73
pecan	135
plain	85
wholewheat	89
Panettone, 1 slice	322
Paper-wrapped Chicken, Chinese-style, 1 piece	98
Parsley sauce, 1 Tbsp	22
Parsnips, roasted	211
Pashka	300
Pastitsio	820
Pâté	
de Campagne	584
de Canard	1,076
de Foie Gras	648
de Poisson au Asperges	478
Peach	
cardinal	230

cobbler	500
Melba	354
Peanut brittle, 1 piece	77
Peanut butter cookies, 1 piece	70
Pea pods with water chestnuts	307
Pea pods with mushrooms	261
Pear Helene	602
Peking custard	464
Penuche, 1 piece	41
Pepper, Greek stuffed green	120
Pepper, Greek stuffed with rice	160
Peppermint sauce, 1 Tbsp	46
Pepperoni, 1 slice	26
Pfeffernusse, 1 piece	82
Picadillo	400
Piccalilli, 1 Tbsp	12
Pie	
Apple, country	410
Apple, deep dish	445
Banana Cream	626
Blueberry	475
Boston Cream	265
Chocolate cream	610
Coconut cream	462
Coconut custard	400
Key Lime	693
Lemon Meringue	545
Nesselrode	516
Peach	400
Pecan	585

Pumpkin	400
Shoofly	528
Pigeon Pie	587
Pig's feet, 1 foot	251
Pigs in blanket	200
Pilaf	
Bulgur	306
Lamb	572
Rice	312
Piquante sauce, 1 Tbsp	19
Pirog, Beef and Mushroom	727
Piroshki	155
Pissaladiere	474
Pita bread	247
Pizza, 1 slice	
Plain	450
Green peppers	452
Mushrooms	462
Pepperoni	587
Plantains	136
Plum pudding, Steamed	451
Plum sauce, 1 Tbsp	30
Polenta	88
Pollo en Salsa verde	244
Pollo molé verde	367
Popcorn balls, 1 ball	249
Poppy seed bread sticks, 1 piece	18
Pork	
Balls, steamed, Chinese-style	488
Barbecued	357

Barbecued with vegetables, Chinese-style	640
Breaded, Italian-style	423
Choucroute garnie	1,000
with rice, Spanish-style	481
Crown roast	584
Loin, stuffed with apples and prunes	685
Lo mein	849
Red, cooked with chestnuts, Chinese-style	432
Sliced, Chinese-style	306
Sliced with green pepper, Chinese-style	411
Soong	666
Spareribs, barbecued	415
Spareribs, Chinese	555
Stuffed with oysters	400
Subgum chow mein	322
Suckling pig	1,100
Sweet and sour, Chinese-style	643
Sweet and sour stew	629
Szechuan-style with bean curd	576
Tenderloin, roast	345
Twice cooked in brown sauce	625
Twice cooked in Hoisin sauce	548
Teriyaki	453
Portugese Filhos, 1 piece	45
Potato Bread, 1 slice	70
Potatoes	
Anna	186
Au Gratin	310
Dauphine	268
Duchess	209

French-fried	232
Hash Brown	230
Lyonnaise	289
Pancakes	144
Potage Saint-Germain	102
Rosti	162
Salad	475
Salad, German-style	270
Scalloped	215
Pot-au-feu	547
Poulet	
a l'Estragon	435
Bonne Femme	410
Cordon Bleu	502
Roti Chasseur	428
Roti Normande	463
Pound Cake, 1 slice	363
Pralines, 1 piece	173
Profiteroles, 1 piece	97
Prosciutto and melon	120
Pudding	
Bread and butter	258
Chocolate	312
Indian	374
Plum, steamed	442
Rice	255
Tapioca	220
Pumpernickel Bread, 1 slice	84
Quenelles, Chicken	493
Fish	148

Saltimbocca   520
Sandwiches
  Bacon, lettuce, and tomato   268
  Bagel with cream cheese   255
  Bagel with lox and cream cheese   355
  Bologna   355
  Cheese, grilled   400
  Cheese, grilled with bacon   543
  Cheese, grilled with tomato   415
  Chopped liver   382
  Corned beef   446
  Fried egg   225
  Lobster salad   255
  Meatball with tomato sauce   400
  Meatloaf   300
  Monte Cristo   920
  Pastrami   560
  Roast beef, overstuffed   490
  Reuben   582
  Salami   394
  Shrimp salad   250
  Steak   353
  Tongue, overstuffed   475
  Tuna fish salad   324
  Turkey club   505
Sangria   93
Sardine Fraiches Marines, 4 oz   328
Sashimi, assorted, 4 oz   100
  tako, 4 oz   87
Sate   500

Sauce Supreme, 1 Tbsp ... 34
Saucisson rémoulade ... 631
Sauerbraten ... 570
Sauerkraut, with juniper berries, braised ... 257
   with caraway seeds ... 72
Sausage and Peppers, 2 pieces ... 882
Scallops, broiled ... 210
   en Brochette ... 254
Scampi ... 178
Scrapple ... 288
Scungilli marinara ... 269
Sfogliatelli ... 244
Shabu-shabu ... 448
Shepherd's Pie ... 500
Shish kebab ... 679
Shortbread, Scottish ... 152
Shortcake, strawberry ... 591
Shrimp
   Ajillo, 8 large ... 466
   in almond sauce, 8 large ... 333
   Balls, Chinese-style ... 286
   Batter-fried, Chinese-style, 1 piece ... 84
   with bean curd, 12 medium ... 980
   with black bean sauce, Chinese-style ... 464
   Braised, Chinese-style 12 medium ... 905
   Butterfly, Japanese-style ... 250
   with cashews ... 536
   creole ... 344
   Egg foo yong ... 356
   Fried in shell, Chinese-style, 12 medium ... 674

Clam chowder, New England	283
Chicken noodle	78
Chicken and rice	78
Chicken with bean curd, Japanese-style	74
Consommé	42
Escarole	138
Garlic	197
Gazpacho	192
Hungarian cherry	375
Hungarian cream of barley	204
Minestrone	243
Miso with bean curd	79
Miso with fish balls	142
Mulligatawny	304
Mushroom, cream of	272
Oxtail	329
Pastina	134
Peanut, cream of	520
Potato	209
Pumpkin	150
Sauerkraut	128
Senegalese	314
Stracciatelli	125
Stschy	167
Tortellini	210
Turtle, home style	278
Vegetable, cream of	340
Sour cream and chive, 1 Tbsp	29
Sour Dough Bread, 1 slice	65
Souvlaki	291

Spaghetti, 1 cup

Alfredo	405
Bolognese	357
with butter, cream and parmesan	401
Carbonara	860
Clam sauce, red	300
Clam sauce, white	344
Fagioli	348
with meatballs in sauce	853
Paglia e fieno	506
al pesto	980
Pomodoro	268
with sausage	471
Spatzle	165
Spiedini with anchovy	386
Spinach au gratin	275
Spinach, creamed	144
Spoon bread	632
Spumoni, 1 cup	510
Squid, Mediterranean	390
Stuffed with Rice, Greek-style	354
Squirrel Stew	500
Steamed Chinese sausage	778
Steamed Scallops with cabbage, Chinese-style, 8 pieces	300
Steamed Whole Fish, Chinese-style, 1 lb	902
Stifado	228
Stollen, 1 slice	145
Strawberries Romanoff	322
Strawberry Shortcake	500

Strudel
Almond	398
Apple	360
Cheese	410
Cherry	405
Poppy seed	400

Stuffing, 1 cup
Chestnut and mushroom	472
Corn bread	700
Herbed	210
Rice	263
Sage and onion	220

Submarine, 1 roll	381
Sukiyaki	348

Sushi
Chirashi	460
Norimaki	468
Tekka maki	400

Sweet and Sour Chinese meatballs	936
Sweet and Sour fish, 1 lb	902
Sweet and Sour sauce, 1 Tbsp	20
Tabbouleh	304

Tacos
Bean	275
Cheese	205
Chicken	245
Chili	348
Chorizo	367

Taffy, 1 piece	50
Tahini sauce, ¼ cup	167

Tamale pie	268
Tandoori fish	300
Shrimp, 10–12	288
Taramasalata, 1 Tbsp	100
Tartar sauce, 1 Tbsp	92
Tarte au champignon	382
au Oignons	570
Tea Eggs, 1 egg	85
Tempura	590
Tempura sauce, 1 Tbsp	5
Teriyaki	
Beef	213
Chicken	380
Pork	462
Teriyaki sauce, 1 Tbsp	15
Toad in the Hole	700
Toast, French, 1 slice	143
Toll House Cookies, 1 piece	60
Tomato Aspic	73
Tomatos, broiled	126
Tomato sauce, 1 Tbsp	10
Bolognese, 1 cup	330
Italian-style, 1 cup	215
with red clam, 1 cup	300
Tomatos, stewed	43
Tortellini with butter and parmesan	582
with ricotta and cream	600
Tortillas, 1 piece, plain	75
Chili	196
Chorizo	500

Sweetbreads

braised	300
creamed	535
with mushrooms	575
sauteed	200
with sherry	585
Terrine of Veal and Ham	250
Vitello Tonnata	850
a la zingara	602
Venison Burgers	360
Ragout of	437
Roast saddle of	205
Vichyssoise	410
Vinaigrette, 1 Tbsp	100
Weiner Schnitzel	415
a la Holstein	457
White sauce, 1 cup	400
Wild Boar, pot roast	500
Wild Duck, roasted	265
Won ton, fried sweet, 1 piece	59
Yakinasu, 4 oz	38
Yakitori	263
Yakitori donburi	781
Yam, candied	315
Yankee pot roast	775
Yogurt kholodnyk	40
Yogurt sauce, 1 Tbsp	9
Yorkshire Pudding	78
Yorkshire Scones, 1 piece	150
Yudofu	83

Zabaglione	177
Zeppole, 1 piece	42
Zucchini, Fried, 1 strip	37
Italian style	100
Sautéed, ½ cup	71
Zuppa di pesce	458
Zuppa Inglese	378

FROZEN DINNERS,

1 complete dinner (see also pp 141-144 and pp 150-153)

Beans and Franks	
Banquet	591
Morton	530
Swanson	550
Beef	
Banquet	312
Chopped	443
La Choy	342
Lean Cuisine Oriental	280
Morton	270
Chopped	340

Country Table	540
Steak House	920
Swanson	370
3-Course	490
Chopped	460
Hungry Man	540
Hungry Man 18 oz	730
Weight Watchers 10 oz	387
Weight Watchers 16 oz	586
Beef and Beans	
Swanson	500
Beef Stroganoff	
Stouffer's	390
Chicken	
La Choy	354
Morton	240
Swanson boneless	730
Weight Watchers	330
Chicken and Biscuits	
Green Giant	200
Chicken Croquettes	
Morton	410
Chicken Cacciatore	
Stouffer's	313
Weight Watchers	356
Chicken and Dumplings	
Banquet	282
Morton	280
Chicken, fried	
Banquet	530

Man Pleaser	1,026
Morton	470
Country Table	710
Swanson	570
3-Course	630
Hungry Man	620
Hungry Man, 15¼ oz	910
Hungry Man, Barbecue	760
Crispy Fried	650
Chicken, glazed	
Lean Cuisine	270
Chicken with noodles	
Morton	260
Chicken, oriental	
Weight Watchers	320
Chicken Parmigiana and Spinach	
Weight Watchers	200
Chicken and vegetables	
Lean Cuisine	260
Chop Suey	
Banquet	282
Chow Mein	
Banquet	282
Green Giant	130
Lean Cuisine	240
Enchilada	
Banquet	
Beef	479
Cheese	459
El Chico	680

Swanson	570
Van de Kamp	
Beef	420
Cheese	430
Fish	
Banquet	382
Haddock	419
Perch	434
Lean Cuisine	200
Morton	270
Weight Watchers	
Flounder	240
Haddock	250
Perch	320
Sole	240
Turbot	490
Fish and Chips	
Swanson	450
Hungry Man	760
Ham	
Banquet	369
Morton	440
Swanson	380
Hash	
Banquet	372
Italian	
Banquet	446
Swanson	420
Lasagna	
Lean Cuisine Zucchini Lasagne	260

Lean Line	270
Swanson	740
Macaroni and beef	
Banquet	394
Morton	260
Swanson	400
Macaroni and cheese	
Banquet	326
Morton	320
Swanson	390
Manicotti	
Lean Line	270
Meat Loaf	
Banquet	412
Morton	340
Country Table	480
Swanson	530
Meatball	
Swanson	400
Mexican	
Banquet	571
Combination	571
El Chico	820
Swanson	600
Pepper	
La Choy	349
Polynesian	
Swanson	490
Pork	
Swanson	470

Queso
El Chico 810
Salisbury Steak
Banquet 390
Morton 290
Country Table 430
Swanson 790
3-Course 490
Hungry Man 870
Saltillo
El Chico 790
Sausage with veal, 1 link
Lean Line 90
Stuffed Shells
Lean Line 260
Shrimp
La Choy 325
Spaghetti with beef
Lean Cuisine 280
Spaghetti and meatball
Banquet 450
Morton 360
Swanson 410
Hungry Man 660
Swiss Steak
Swanson 350
Tacos, beef
El Chico 410
Turkey
Banquet 293

Man Pleaser	620
Morton	350
Country Table	600
Swanson	360
3-Course	520
Hungry Man	740
Weight Watchers	400
Veal Parmigiana	
Banquet	421
Morton	330
Swanson	520
Hungry Man	910
Weight Watchers	230
Western	
Banquet	417
Morton	410
Swanson	460
Hungry Man	890
Ziti, baked	
Lean Line	270

CHAPTER 15

Fingertip Low Calorie Guide

OVER 350 CALORIES

Frozen entrees (at less than 30 calories per ounce)

Banquet Buffet Supper Beef and Noodles, 32 oz	754
Banquet Buffet Supper Beef Stew, 32 oz	700
Banquet Buffet Supper Chicken and Noodles, 32 oz	764
Banquet Buffet Supper Beef sliced with gravy, 32 oz	782
Banquet Buffet Supper Turkey, 32 oz	564
La Choy Chicken	354

15

Morton Country Table Salisbury Steak, 15 oz   430
Swanson Hungry-Man Turkey, 13¼ oz   380
Weight Watchers Turkey Tetrazzini, 13 oz   380

200-350 CALORIES

Frozen entrees (at less than 30 calories per ounce)

Beef
  Banquet, 11 oz   312
  Lean Cuisine, 9⅛ oz   280
  Morton, 10 oz   270
Chicken
  Morton, 10 oz   240
  Stouffer's
    Chicken a la King, 9½ oz   330
    Creamed Chicken, 6½ oz   300
    Chicken Divan, 8½ oz   335
  Weight Watchers, 15 oz   330
Chicken and Biscuits
  Green Giant, 7 oz   200
Chicken Creole
  Weight Watchers, 13 oz   250
Chicken and Dumplings
  Banquet, 12 oz   282
  Morton, 11 oz   280

Chicken with Noodles
Green Giant, 9 oz   250
Morton, 10½ oz   260

Chicken Oriental
Weight Watchers, 16 oz   320

Chicken Parmigiana and Spinach
Weight Watchers, 9 oz   200

Chicken and Vegetables
Lean Cuisine, 12¾ oz   260

Chicken White Meat with Peas
Weight Watchers, 9 oz   270

Chop Suey
Banquet, 12 oz   282

Chow Mein
Banquet, 12 oz   282
Lean Cuisine, 11¼ oz   240

Eggplant Parmigiana
Weight Watchers, 13 oz   280

Fish
Lean Cuisine, 9 oz   200
Morton, 9 oz   270
Weight Watchers
   Flounder, 16 oz   240
   Haddock, 16 oz   250
   Perch, 16 oz   320
   Sole, 16 oz   240
   Sole with peas, mushrooms and
     lobster sauce, 9½ oz   200

Green Peppers with Beef
Green Giant, 7 oz   200

15

Lasagne
Lean Line, 10 oz   270
Lasagne, Zucchini
Lean Cuisine, 11 oz   260
Macaroni with Beef
Green Giant, 9 oz   240
Morton, 10 oz   260
Macaroni and Cheese
Banquet, 12 oz   326
Morton, 11 oz   320
Manicotti
Lean Line, 11 oz   270
Salisbury Steak
Banquet, 11 oz   390
Morton, 11 oz   290
Shells, Stuffed
Lean Line, 11 oz   260
Spaghetti with Beef
Lean Cuisine, 11½ oz   280
Turkey
Banquet, 11 oz   293
Swanson Turkey Slices, 8¾ oz   260
Ziti, Baked
Lean Line, 10 oz   270
Ziti with Veal and sauce
Weight Watchers, 13 oz   350
Veal Parmigiana with Zucchini
Weight Watchers, 9½ oz   230

Canned Entrees (at less than 30 calories per ounce)

Pasta, one can
Ravioli
Franco-American Beef, 7½ oz   220
Rotini
Franco-American, 7½ oz   200
Macaroni
Franco-American, 7½ oz   220
Macaroni and Meatballs
Franco-American, 7½ oz   220
Meat, one can
Beef Goulash
Hormel, 7½ oz   240
Ham, whole
Hormel, 6 oz   312
Tuna, in water, drained
Chicken of the Sea solid white, 7 oz can   216

Fish, Fresh

Crab, steamed, meat only, 8 oz   211
Haddock, fillets, 8 oz   180
Halibut, fillets, 8 oz   226
Oysters, Pacific and Western, meat only, 8 oz   207

15

Meat

Beef

Chuck

boneless, lean only, braised, 4 oz	219
boneless, lean only, stewed, 4 oz	243
Flank steak, boneless, all lean, braised, 4 oz	222
ground, lean with 10% fat, 4 oz	203
porterhouse steak with 9% bone, lean only, broiled, 4 oz without bone	254
round steak, boneless, lean only, braised or broiled, 4 oz	296
sirloin steak, 7% bone, lean only, broiled, 4 oz without bone	235
T-bone, 11% bone, lean only, broiled, 4 oz without bone	253

Ham

fresh, lean only

baked, without bone and skin, 4 oz	246

light cured, lean only

baked, without bone and skin, 4 oz	328

Lamb

Leg, lean only, roasted, boneless, 4 oz	211
loin chops, with bone, lean only, broiled, 4 oz	213
rib chops, with bone, lean only, broiled, 4 oz	239
shoulder, lean only, roasted, boneless, 4 oz	233

Pork
Picnic, without bone and skin, lean only, baked
or roasted, 4 oz   239

Veal
loin cuts, lean with fat, braised or broiled,
without bone, 4 oz   245
round with rump (roasts and leg cutlets),
lean with fat, braised or broiled, without
bone, 4 oz   245

Poultry

Chicken
roasted, without skin, 4 oz   204
stewed, light meat without skin, 4 oz   207
Turkey, roasted, light meat without skin, 4 oz   200

101-200 CALORIES

Pasta

All pasta, dry, one cup
cooked till tender, (approx)   190
cooked till firm, (approx)   155

Canned, 1 can

Franco-American macaroni and cheese, 7½ oz   184

Franco-American spaghetti with cheese, 7⅜ oz   170

Franco-American spaghetti with cheese
sauce, 7⅜ oz   160

Meat Entrees (at less than 30 calories per ounce)

Frozen

Beef, chipped, creamed
  Banquet, 5 oz   124

Beef, sliced
  Banquet, barbecue sauce, 5 oz   126
  Banquet, with gravy, 5 oz   116
  Green Giant, 5 oz   130

Beef Stew
  Green Giant Boil-in-Bag, 9 oz   160
  Green Giant, with biscuits, 7 oz   190

Veal steaks
  Hormel, 4 oz   130

Meat Entrees, canned (at less than 30 calories per ounce), 1 can

Beef, corned with cabbage
   Hormel, 8 oz   150
Beef stew
   Dinty Moore, 7½ oz   184
   Swanson, 7½ oz   190
Pork, sliced, with gravy
   Morton House, 6¼ oz   190

Poultry entrees

Frozen (at less than 30 calories per ounce)
   Chicken a la King
      Banquet, 5 oz   138
Canned, 1 can
   Chicken stew
      Swanson, 7½ oz   180
   Turkey slices
      Morton House, 6¼ oz   140
   Chicken, fresh
      Broiled, meat only, 4 oz   154

Seafood

Clams, canned, drained, 1 can
   Doxsee, 8 oz   112
   Doxsee, 12 oz   147
Shrimp marinara, with shells, frozen
   Buitoni, 4 oz   116

Fish, fresh, 4 oz, meat only

Abalone	111
Black Sea Bass	106
Butterfish, gulf	108
Catfish, fresh water	117
Croaker, Atlantic	109
Lake Herring (Cisco)	109
Lobster	109
Mussels	108
Ocean Pearch, Pacific	108
Red or Grey Snapper	106
Sea bass, white	109
Shrimp	103
Sturgeon	107
Tautog (Blackfish)	101

51-100 CALORIES

Miscellaneous

Pabst Extra Light Beer	70
Whipped butter, 1 Tbsp	65
Farina, *Pillsbury*, ⅔ cup	80
Grits, *Quaker* Instant, 1 packet	79
One Egg, raw or boiled	
extra large	94
large	82
medium	72
Canned Spaghetti with meatballs, *Libby's*, 1 cup	84
Canned Spanish rice, *Libby's*, 1 cup	57

Chinese dishes

Chow mein, canned, 1 cup	
La Choy	
beef	72
chicken	68
mushroom	85
pepper	89
shrimp	61
Chow mein, frozen	
Banquet, 1 bag	89

La Choy beef, 1 cup	97
La Choy shrimp, 1 cup	73
Pea pods, frozen, 1 package	
La Choy	90
Won Ton, frozen, 1 cup	
La Choy	92

Dairy

Cottage Cheese, low fat, ½ cup	
Borden	90
Breakstone	90
Friendship	100
Lucerne	100
Viva	100
Weight Watchers	90
Milk, 8 ounces	
Buttermilk	
.1% fat *Borden*	88
.2% fat *Sealtest* skim	71
.5% fat *Borden*	90
.8% fat *Golden Nugget*	92
.8% fat *Light 'n Lively*	95
Dry, non-fat milk, reconstituted	81
Skin or low-fat	
no fat *Lucerne*	90
.1% fat *Borden*	81

fortified	81
.1% fat *Sealtest*	79
Yogurt, plain, ½ cup	
Borden Lite-Line lowfat	70
Sealtest Light 'n Lively lowfat	70
Danny On-A-Stick, uncoated	65

Meat, canned

Beef stew	
Libby's, 1 cup	78
Ham, whole	
Wilson's certified boned and rolled, 1 oz	56

Poultry

Chicken stew with dumplings, canned	
Libby's, 1 cup	88
Turkey with gravy, frozen	
Banquet, 5 oz	98
Green Giant, 5 oz	100

Seafood, canned

Clams
Snow's, ½ cup	60
Sau-Sea, 4 oz	99

Gefilte Fish
Manischewitz, 3 oz piece	53
Manischewitz whitefish and pike, 3 oz piece	64
Mother's, 4 oz piece	55

Oysters
Bumblebee, ½ cup	86

Shrimp
Bumblebee, 4½ oz can	90

Seafood, fresh, meat only, 4 oz

Clams	92
Cod	88
Crayfish	82
Croaker, white	95
Flounder	89
Ocean Perch, Atlantic	100
Oysters	75
Pickerel	95
Pike	100
Sand Dab	89
Sauger	95
Scallops	92
Sole	90
Squid	95
Tilefish	90

Fruits and Vegetables

Artichokes
boiled, drained, 1 whole bud   67
Beets
raw, diced, 1 cup   58
Broccoli
boiled, drained, 8 oz   59
Carrots
raw, slices, 1 cup   53
Chayote
raw, 1 medium squash   56
Cranberries
fresh, without stems, 1 cup   52
Currants, red or white
trimmed, 1 cup   55
Dock or Sorrel
raw with stems, 1 lb   89
Endive, French or Belgian
trimmed, 1 lb   68
Escarole
untrimmed, 1 lb   80
Grapefruit
pink or red, with seeds
    whole, with skin, 1 lb   87
    sections, 1 cup   80
pink or red, seedless
    whole, with skin, 1 lb   93
    sections, 1 cup   80

white, with seeds
  whole, with skin, 1 lb 84
  sections, 1 cup 82
white, seedless
  whole, with skin, 1 lb 87
  sections, 1 cup 78

Honeydew Melon
whole, with rinds and seeds, 1 lb 94
cubed or diced, 1 cup 56

Lettuce
Iceberg
  whole, 1 lb 56
Loose Leaf
  whole, 1 lb 52
Romaine or cos
  whole, 1 lb 52

Pawpaw
peeled and seeded, 4 oz 96

Papaya
peeled and seeded, cubed, 1 cup 55

Peaches
pared, sliced, 1 cup 65

Raspberries
black, 1 cup 98
red, 1 cup 70

Strawberries
whole, 1 cup 55

Watermelon
whole, with rind, 1 lb 54

20-50 CALORIES

Breads, Buns and Rolls

Bread, 1 slice
Gluten
  Thomas   32
Protein
  Thomas   45
Rice Cakes
  Spiral   36
Wheat
  Thomas   50
White
  Arnold Melba Thin   40
  Fresh Horizons   50
  Pepperidge Farm Very Thin   40
  Weight Watchers   35
Buns and Rolls, 1 piece
  Pepperidge Farm Old-Fashioned   37
  Pepperidge Farm Party   35
Margarine, 1 Tbsp
  Blue Bonnet Diet   50
  Fleischmann Diet   50
  Imitation   50

15

Candy, 1 piece

Rolo	28

Cheese, 1 oz

Farmer's	
Friendship	38
Ricotta	
Borden	42
Imitation Cream Cheese	
Philadelphia	50
American, grated	
Borden	30

Chinese Dishes

Apple-Cinnamon roll, frozen	
La Choy, 1 piece	38
Bamboo Shoots, canned	
La Choy, 8 oz	23
Bean sprouts, canned	
La Choy, 8 oz	24
Chow Mein, canned, 1 cup	
Chun King	44
La Choy, meatless	47

Egg Rolls, frozen
   La Choy chicken, 1 piece   30
   La Choy lobster, 1 piece   27
Mixed vegetables, canned
   La Choy, 1 cup   35

Cream

Half & Half, 1 Tbsp   20
   Lucerne Real Cream topping, 1 whipped oz   20

Dips, 1 oz

Bean, Jalapeño
   Frito-Lay   36
   Gebhardt   30
   Granny Goose   37
   Lucerne   36
Clam
   Lucerne   34
Gelatin
   Knox gelatin, 1 envelope   28
Gravy
   French's Pork, mix, ½ cup   40

15

Jelly, 1 Tbsp

Apple
  Kraft, Low Calorie   22
  Diet Delight   22
Apricot Pineapple Jam
  Diet Delight   21
Blackberry Apple
  Kraft, low calorie   22
Blackberry Jam
  Diet Delight   21
Grape
  Kraft, Low Calorie   22
  Diet Delight   21
Raspberry Jam
  Diet Delight   21

Meat, 1 oz, canned

Beef
  Corned, canned
    Safeway   35
  Dried
    Swift   42
  Smoked
    Safeway   35
    Safeway spicy   40

Beef roast
  Wilson   33
Ham
  Wilson certified fully cooked   48
  Wilson certified *Tender Made*   44
  Wilson certified festival ham   48
Pastrami
  Safeway   40
Scrapple
  Oscar Mayer in tube   50
  Oscar Mayer Philadelphia style   45

Olives

Green, 10 large   45
Manzanillo Black, 10 large   50

Popcorn, 1 cup

Pops-Rite, popped   38
Wise, cheese-flavored, ready to eat   49

15

Poultry

Safeway smoked chicken, 1 oz	50
Safeway smoked turkey, 1 oz	50

Pudding, ½ cup

D-Zerta

butterscotch	25
chocolate	20
vanilla	30

Salad Dressing, 1 Tbsp

French

Ann Page Low Calorie	25
Kraft Low Calorie	25
Nu Made Low Calorie	20

Italian

Wish-Bone Low Calorie	20

May Lo Naise

Tillie Lewis	25

Russian

Wish-Bone Low Calorie	25

Thousand Island
  Ann Page Low Calorie   25
  Wish-Bone Low Calorie   25
Whipped
  Tillie Lewis   25

Sauces & Spreads

Crosse & Blackwell Anchovy Paste 1 Tbsp   20
Hunt's Tomato Sauce, 4 oz   35
  with mushrooms, 4 oz   40
Open Pit Barbecue, 1 Tbsp   26

Vegetables, canned and frozen

Artichoke Hearts
  Birds Eye, 3 oz   20
Asparagus, 1 cup, canned
  cuts   40
  spears   40
  spears and tips   35
  whole   50
Asparagus, frozen
  Birds Eye, 3.3 oz   25
  Seabrook Farms, ½ cup   23

15

Beans, green canned, 1 cup
french

Del Monte	40
Green Giant	30
Kounty Kist	40
Libby's	35

whole

Del Monte	35
Green Giant	30
Kounty Kist	40
Libby's	35
Stokely-Van Camp	40

Beans, green, frozen

Birds Eye, 3.3 oz	25
Kounty Kist, 1 cup	30
Seabrook Farms, 1 cup	42

Beans, wax or yellow, 1 cup

Del Monte	35
Libby's	40
Stokely-Van Camp	45

Broccoli, frozen

Birds Eye 3.3 oz	25
Green Giant, 1 cup	30
Kounty Kist, 1 cup	30
Seabrook Farms, 1 cup	46

Brussels Sprouts, frozen

Birds Eye, 3.3 oz	30
Green Giant, 1 cup	50
Kounty Kist, 1 cup	50

Carrots, canned, 1 cup
  Libby's   40
  S & W   44
Cauliflower, frozen
  Birds Eye 3.3 oz   25
  Green Giant, 1 cup   25
  Kounty Kist, 1 cup   25
Collard Greens
  Birds Eye, 3.3 oz   30
  Seabrook Farms, 1 cup   44
Mixed Vegetables
  Kounty Kist, California, 1 cup   30
Mustard Greens
  Seabrook Farms, ½ cup   21
Sauerkraut, canned, 1 cup   50
Spinach, canned, 1 cup   45
Spinach, frozen, 1 cup   50
Tomatoes, canned
  Hunt's stewed, 4 oz   30
  Libby's whole, 1 cup   45
  S & W whole, 1 cup   42
  Stokely-Van Camp, whole   50
  Townhouse, whole   50
Turnip Greens
  Birds Eye 3.3 oz   20
  Seabrook Farms, ½ cup   22
  Stokely-Van Camp, ½ cup   22

Fruits and Vegetables, fresh, 1 cup unless noted

Asparagus	
cut spears	35
Bamboo shoots	
cuts	41
Bean Sprouts	37
Beans, green or snap	
cuts	34
Beans, wax or yellow	
cuts	30
Beet Greens	26
Cabbage, red or green, chopped	22
Cantelope, cubed	48
Casaba Melon, cubed	45
Cauliflower, flowerets	27
Swiss Chard, leaves only	32
Eggplant, diced	50
Radish, diced	20
Rhubarb, raw diced	20
Summer Squash, diced	35
Tomatos, sliced	40
Turnips, cubed	39

Fruit and Vegetable drinks, 6 oz

Cranberry	
Ocean Spray low calorie	35

Cranberry apple
   Ocean Spray cranapple low calorie   30
Sauerkraut
   Libby's   20
Tomato
   Campbell's   35
   Del Monte   35
   Heinz   38
   Hunt's   43
   Libby's   39
   S & W   22
   Sacramento   35
   Stokely-Van Camp   33
   Townhouse   35
   Welch's   38
Tomato cocktail
   Ortega Snap-E-Tom   38
Vegetable cocktail
   S & W   21
   Townhouse   35
   V-8   35

UNDER 20 CALORIES

Beverages

Note: virtually all sodas that are called *low-calorie*, *sugar-free* or *dietetic* contain 2 calories or less.

Bouillon, 1 cube

Beef
Herb-Ox	6
Maggi	6
Wyler's	7
Wyler's Instant	10

Chicken
Herb-Ox	6
Maggi	7
Wyler's	8
Wyler's Instant	6

Onion
Herb-Ox	10
Wyler's	6

Vegetable
Herb-Ox	6
Wyler's	6

Breath Mints, 1 piece

Certs clear	8
Certs pressed	6
Chewels	10
Clorets mints	6
Dentyne dynamints	2
Lifesavers	7
Trident mints	8

Broth, 1 packet

Herb-Ox
Beef	8
Chicken	12
Onion	14
Vegetable	12

Candy, Dietetic

Estee, 1 piece
chocolate covered raisins	6
gum drops	3
hard candies	12
mint candies	4

Cocktail Mix, non-alcoholic, 1 oz

Holland House Bloody Mary	6
Holland House Whiskey Sour	9

Coffee, 1 cup

ground	2
instant	4

15

Condiments, 1 Tbsp

A-1 sauce	12
Catsup	
Del Monte	15
Chili sauce	
Heinz	17
Horseradish	2
Mustard	
French's Brown	15
French's Yellow	16
Grey Poupon Dijon	15
Soy sauce	
La Choy	8
Taco sauce	
Old El Paso	4
Vinegar	1
Worcestershire	10

Cookies, 1 piece

Angel Puffs	
Stella D'Oro Dietetic	17
Arrowroot	
Sunshine	16
Royal Nuggets	
Stella D'Oro	1

Vanilla Snaps
  Nabisco   13
Vanilla Wafers
  Sunshine   15
  Nabisco   18
Zuzu Ginger Snaps
  Nabisco   16

Cough Drops   9

Crackers, 1 cracker

Cheez-It
  Sunshine   6
Cheeze
  Keebler   11
Flings Curls
  Nabisco   10
Matzos
  Manischewitz Tam Tams   14
Melba Toast
  Old London
    Garlic   9
    Onion   10
    Pumpernickel   17
    Rye   17
    Sesame   10
    Wheat   17
    White   17

15

Oyster
Keebler   3
Sunshine   3
Ritz
Nabisco   16
Saltines
Keebler Zesta   12
Nabisco Premium   12
Sunshine Krispy   11
Sociables
Nabisco   10
Triangle Thins
Nabisco   8
Wheat Thins
Nabisco   9

Creamers, Non-Dairy, 1 tsp

Coffee-Mate, Carnation, 1 pkt   11
Coffee-Tone   12
Cremora, Pet   11

Gelatin, mix, ½ cup

D-Zerta   8
Royal Sweet As You Please   6

Gravy, ¼ cup, mix

Au Jus
Durkee	8
French's	8
McCormick	4
Schilling	4

Brown
Durkee	15
Durkee with mushrooms	15
Durkee with onions	17
McCormick Lite	10
Weight Watchers	8
with mushrooms	12
with onions	13

Chicken
Durkee home style	18
McCormick Lite	10
Pillsbury home style	15
Schilling Lite	10
Weight Watchers	10

Mushroom
McCormick	19
Schilling	19

Pork
Durkee	18

Mushroom Steak
Dawn Fresh	4

Swiss Steak
Durkee	11

15

Gum, 1 piece

Adams	9
Beeman	10
Beech-Nut	9
Beechies	6
Black Jack	9
Care Free	8
Chiclets	6
Clorets	6
Clove	5
Dentyne	5
Estee	3
Freshen-Up	9
Fruit Stripe	9
Orbit	8
Trident	5
Wrigley's	10

Jelly, 1 tsp

Ann Page, all flavors	18
Diet Delight Strawberry	18
Kraft, all flavors	16
S & W, all flavors	10
Smuckers Slenderella, all flavors	8

Oil

Pam Vegetable spray	7

Pickles

Capers, 1 Tbsp
Crosse & Blackwell	6

Onions, cocktail, 1 Tbsp
Crosse & Blackwell	1

Peppers, 1 oz
Chile Green, *Ortega*	5
Hot Pickled, *Old El Paso*	9

Dill Pickles, spears, 1 piece
Bond's	2
Del Monte	7
Heinz	7
Smucker's	8

Sour Pickles, 1 piece
Del Monte	10

Salad dressings, 1 Tbsp

Blue Cheese
Ann Page Low Calorie	18
Kraft Low Calorie	14

Tillie Lewis   12
Weight Watchers   10

Caesar
Pfeiffer Low Calorie   10

French
Pfeiffer Low Calorie   18
Weight Watchers   4
Tillie Lewis   12

Italian
Ann Page Low Calorie   14
Kraft Low Calorie   6
Nu Made Low Calorie   16
Pfeiffer Low Calorie   10
Tillie Lewis   6
Weight Watchers   2

Red Wine
Pfeiffer Low Calorie   10

Russian
Pfeiffer Low Calorie   15
Tillie Lewis   12
Weight Watchers   12

Thousand Island
Pfeiffer Low Calorie   15
Tillie Lewis   18
Weight Watchers   12

Sauces, 1 Tbsp

Barbecue
  French's — 14
Enchilada
  Old El Paso hot — 9
  Old El Paso mild — 10
Lemon-Butter
  Weight Watchers — 8

Sugar, 1 tsp — 15

Pancake Syrup, 1 Tbsp

Cary's Diet — 10
Diet Delight — 15
S & W — 12
Tillie Lewis — 14

Tea, 1 cup — 1

lemon-flavored
  Nestea — 2

Toppings, 1 Tbsp

No-Cal
all flavors except chocolate and coffee	0
No-Cal chocolate & coffee	6

whipped mix
D-Zerta	8
Dream Whip	10

Vegetables and Fruits, Fresh

Cabbage
Chinese, cuts, 1 cup	11
spoon (Bakchoy), cuts, 1 cup	11

Celery
1 large outer stalk	7
3 small inner stalks	9

Chicory greens
cuts, 1 cup	11
10 inner leaves	5

Endive, French or Belgian
1 head, 5-7"	8
10 small leaves	5
chopped, 1 cup	14

Escarole, cuts, 1 cup	10
Mushrooms, chopped, 1 cup	20
Pepper, sweet, green, sliced, 1 cup	18

Pickles
   dill, 1 large   15
   sour, 1 large   14
Spinach, trimmed and chopped, 1 cup   14
Watercress, 1 cup   7